Do Right by Me

Do Right by Me

Learning to Raise Black Children

in White Spaces

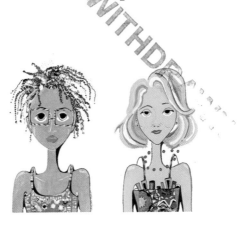

Valerie I. Harrison

and Kathryn Peach D'Angelo

TEMPLE UNIVERSITY PRESS　*Philadelphia* · *Rome* · *Tokyo*

TEMPLE UNIVERSITY PRESS
Philadelphia, Pennsylvania 19122
tupress.temple.edu

Library of Congress Cataloging-in-Publication Data

Names: Harrison, Valerie I., 1962– author. | D'Angelo, Kathryn Peach, 1972–
   author.
Title: Do right by me : learning to raise black children in white spaces /
   Valerie I. Harrison and Kathryn Peach D'Angelo.
Description: Philadelphia : Temple University Press, 2021. | Includes
   bibliographical references and index. | Summary: "This book orients
   parents and communities of black children, including white adoptive
   parents, to the particular challenges and inequalities race brings to
   childhood. The authors present research, insight, and their own
   experience to guide parents to challenges related to education, health,
   safety, self-esteem, and community building"—Provided by publisher.
Identifiers: LCCN 2020013140 (print) | LCCN 2020013141 (ebook) |
   ISBN 9781439919958 (trade paperback) | ISBN 9781439919965 (pdf)
Subjects: LCSH: Interracial adoption—United States. | African American
   children—United States. | Race awareness in children—United States. |
   Adoptive parents—United States. | Adopted children—United States. |
   Racially mixed families—United States. | United States—Race relations.
Classification: LCC HV875.64 .H36 2021 (print) | LCC HV875.64 (ebook) |
   DDC 649/.14508996073—dc23
LC record available at https://lccn.loc.gov/2020013140
LC ebook record available at https://lccn.loc.gov/2020013141

∞ The paper used in this publication meets the requirements of the American
National Standard for Information Sciences—Permanence of Paper for Printed
Library Materials, ANSI Z39.48-1992

Printed in the United States of America

9 8 7 6 5 4 3 2 1

For Gabriel

Contents

Prologue

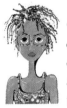 Conversations about race and racism fill homes, classrooms, theaters, and the minds of many Americans, and I have certainly participated in my share. But a very specific event prompted my friend Katie and me to write this book and share our conversation. I am black, and Katie and her husband are white adoptive parents raising their son, Gabriel. Gabriel's biological mother is white, and his biological father is black. Our formal education and experiences have given Katie and me access to information, research, resources, and people that inform our conversations about race and racism. However, after Gabriel's birth in 2011, race and racism were no longer theoretical academic topics of conversation for us. The stakes grew from the two of us trying to understand each other's perspectives to a mother navigating how to equip a child with the perspective that would best serve him as he grew up with a different set of experiences from his parents.

We embarked on this journey to write a book that orients parents and other community members to the ways race and racism will affect a black child's life, and despite that, how to raise and nurture healthy and happy children. Dialogue about racism can be difficult and benefits from a knowledge of history, as well as a vocabulary of ideas and practice. Essential to the task is an understanding of racism and how systems continue to perpetuate privileges and disadvantages that your child will have to navigate in ways that you may never have had to. We also wrestle with the issue of why more people are not working to dismantle those systems. This understanding may lead you to see the world and you and your child's place in it differently. The book will introduce our own experiences and bring in research and expertise from education, psychology, sociology, history, law, African American studies, and other fields to make sense of the questions and obstacles we faced and we expect readers to face. While we hope to guide parents and community members, this book will not proceed like a traditional how-to. Instead, readers will learn how race impacts the way the world interacts with a black child, and the way they as adults can provide their child with the knowledge and awareness to resiliently face these challenges. People raised to believe that their place in society is shaped only by individual merit will learn about the obstacles African Americans have faced and continue to face. If a parent is able to communicate this history, they arm black children with the knowledge that they inherit a history of resistance in the face of structural disadvantage, thereby combating the prejudice that associates blackness with laziness, immorality, and overall inferiority. This knowledge guards a child's confidence and well-being, a goal at the heart of our project. Moreover, anyone raised to believe that U.S. history is a story of continued and sustained racial progress will learn that at each historical moment, race is reinscribed for new disadvantage. It is our hope that this knowledge will motivate readers to take a more active approach to eradicating racism in their own time.

This book also tells a story about developing friendships across races and ethnicities. The common refrain "some of my best friends are black" is real for Katie and me. We have nearly twenty years in. We talk almost every day. We each were one of the handful of supporters sitting in the room as the other defended a doctoral disser-tation. Katie was the person in the room taking notes as surgeons spoke too fast and with terminology too unfamiliar for me to fully grasp how they would remove the cancer from my body, but she got it all down. We share secrets. I am her lawyer, and she is my uncredentialed therapist. And I am not the only one. The D'Angelo dinner table can often include more black people than white. They were married, and Gabe was baptized, by a black priest with whom Mike and Katie have been friends for decades.

We guide you on this journey using both of our voices, each in turn. When one of us presents a new idea, the other will recall a scenario that shows how it works in real life; when one of us remembers a question she faced, the other will jump in with the research and insight to put it into perspective and help you think through it. To help keep the shift in voices straight, we called on an artist friend, Susan Jarvis Ragland, and use her artwork to identify the speaker. Throughout the book, we will identify my voice by introducing it with the same piece of Susan's artwork that was placed at the beginning of this prologue. Look for Katie's pic-ture to indicate her voice. Here is the first shift from me to Katie.

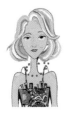 Unlike parents who subscribe to a color-blind or postracial ideology, my husband, Mike, and I confronted head-on the reality that we would need to equip Gabri-el for a life far more complex than anything we had experienced. I learned that I was not alone. Whenever Val encountered white women raising black children (daughters mainly), these women eagerly shared their concerns and questions about everything, from how to care for their daughters' hair and affirm their body image to how to build a diverse community of support. White parents of black children want so badly to parent well and certainly have enough love to go around, yet we have real questions and concerns related to racism, culture, and identity.

Mike and I were clear that we wanted to parent within a village that included people who looked like Gabriel and in a way that prioritized his best interests, but that was not possible without knowing much more than our lives had taught us. That's where this book comes in. Doing right by Gabriel and all black children means learning what disadvantages they will face because of their race, where those disadvantages come from, what effect they have, and how people have been managing them. It's a lesson that many people could benefit from learning. The book is useful not only for white adoptive parents of black children but also for anyone engaged in parenting and nurturing black children, including black or interracial families of origin. The book also provides insights and tools to a broad audience of social scientists, child and family counselors, community organizations, and other educators who engage issues of transracial adoption or child development or who explore current experiences in the areas of social justice and institutionalized racism.

We've organized the book into eight chapters:

Chapter 1. Knowing What You Don't Know: This book is not intended to add new research to the existing studies regarding the efficacy of transracial adoption, but it will make the research that has been done accessible to readers.

Chapter 2. Trapped in History: Understanding the United States' racial history helps explain how our present is structured by racism—to an extent not possible without knowing that history. In order to really open up a conversation about building positive racial identity and navigating racism, participants must first learn the horrific race narrative in the United States and how racist systems continue to impact the lives of black and white people today.

Chapter 3. Too Great for Hope: Perhaps the single most important point of this book is to emphatically show how critical it is for parents of black children, whether adoptive parents or parents of origin, to do everything possible to ensure their children develop a positive racial identity and never feel that they are a failed attempt at being white. This chapter defines positive racial identity and shares tools for getting black children there, covering topics such as African history, culture, art, body image, and spirituality.

Chapter 4. In Living Color: At the heart of it all, our children are guided and shaped by the diverse people that comprise their community. In Chapter 4, Val and I tell a story about developing friendships across races and ethnicities and how absolutely essential that is to raising a child.

 Katie and I then turn to describe how racism plays out in various aspects of a black child's life.

Chapter 5. Black Out: The impact of racism on the health of black people, compounded by racism in the delivery of health care, has created health disparities between black and white Americans that are astounding regardless of income. We share specific steps parents can take to close the gap.

Chapter 6. Not without Education: We hear consistently that education is the "great equalizer." However, in Chapter 6, we scrutinize that assumption and look at the important role of parents to make sure the learning environment is constantly examined and intentionally designed to achieve positive results for children of all races and backgrounds. For example, the chapter explores the research regarding educational outcomes for black children who have at least one black teacher. It also considers data that suggests that black students receive more discipline that results in time out of class than white students for the same behavior. Passive education environments equalize nothing for black children;

a child's community must actively work to make sure that each black child receives the benefits expected by their white peers.

Chapter 7. The Talk: Most often, a child having at least one biological parent of African descent will be regarded by others as black. This is enough for many people to treat that child with fear and prejudice. One does not have to look far into news reports to know that black men and women of all ages are confronted with unconscionable violence simply for being black. This chapter will share resources and tactics parents can use in an effort to help keep their children safe.

Chapter 8. Alchemy of Intention: This final chapter is the culminating expression of what we have grown to know through these chapters. Love is simply not enough. It will take evolutionary consciousness together with an intention to protect, nurture, educate, affirm, encourage, and advocate for every child.

The book's title, *Do Right by Me,* is taken from a line in Alice Walker's prized novel made movie and musical *The Color Purple.* The chief character, Celie, asserts herself after years of abuse from the man she is forced to marry, referred to only as Mister. "Until you do right by me, everything you think about is going to crumble," is her valiant declaration to Mister to end the cycle of abuse. The appeal "do right by me" represents for us the plea of black children for an end to the operation of racist and oppressive systems, policies, and behaviors in their lives today. It is the call that our children charge us with: to take on the responsibility of experiencing discomfort, being brave, and learning uncomfortable truths in order to provide them with a better world.

The name Gabriel turned out to be more predictive of the impact Gabe would have on our community than we could have imagined. In various religious traditions and sacred texts, Gabriel is identified as an archangel who provides clarity by explaining visions and foretelling future events. Our Gabriel has ushered us onto a journey to provide clarity to an area so riddled with misunderstanding and confusion that it continues to divide the world. Even those who profess to be progressive-minded advocates of equity and inclusion may not recognize their blind spots and how their passivity perpetuates the negative impact of racist systems. Gabriel has inspired us to share a conversation that we hope provides greater clarity to anyone concerned about creating a more just and equitable society.

Acknowledgments

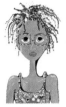This project would not be possible if it were not for a treasured community located in North Central Philadelphia. Known to Philadelphians simply as North Philly, I am grateful for those markers and experiences there that provided inspiration for this project, from the brick row house where my mother grew up near Twenty-First and Dauphin Streets to the beautiful black children I see each day racing across Diamond Street into a school that is woefully underresourced but whose smiles display their hope and resilience. North Philly introduced us to our Temple University family, many of whom are our biggest cheerleaders. It also brought us to the team at Temple Press, who believed in this project even before it fully unfolded.

We would especially like to acknowledge our book editor, Ryan Mulligan. We were an unlikely trio, but you were generous and patient and got us to the finish line. You fueled this work. And to those parents who were not afraid to share their experiences and ask questions, especially Lauren Silver. Thank you.

We are grateful for so many who have encouraged us and provided us with valuable advice. While the people and interactions are far too numerous to mention here, there are those whose support we must specifically acknowledge: Hilary Beard, Darryl DeBreast, Kevin Feeley, Beth Hall, Joseph Harrison, Stephanie Ives, Maya Johnson, Derek Jolly, Tyrell Mann-Barnes, Ali Michael, Grace Osa-Edoh, Catherine Panzarella, Reverend Ricardo Phipps, Erin and Frederick Pratt, Susan Jarvis Ragland, Dina Stonberg, Reverend Stephen D. Thorne, Lily Van Cleave, and Timothy Welbeck. We appreciate you more than you know.

I owe a tremendous debt of gratitude to Molefi K. Asante. I first heard you speak when I was a college student in the 1980s. Your message was new to me. You talked about the need for black people to know themselves, to understand their history, and to feel good about who they were, as well as your belief that this knowledge would help them to do great things. I continue to be in awe of and inspired by your scholarship, courage, and commitment to the liberation of black people everywhere. You planted the seed for this work.

I will always be in the debt of the ancestors, chiefly my parents, Joseph and Frances C. Harrison, for giving me life and love.

And none of this would be possible without God, to whom I am forever grateful.

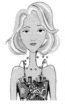 There are several occasions throughout the book where you hear our blended voice as authors, and so much of our gratitude can be expressed on behalf of us both. In addition to these many blessings, I have some more.

To the birth mothers and fathers who have entrusted us with their greatest gift: words will not suffice, so we live every day to do right by our gift.

To my bold and fiercely loving YaYa Sisterhood: there has been no better space to percolate such ideas and wisdom than with you.

As the eldest child of Mary Pat and Charlie Peach, I have been deeply influenced by my parents' humor, resilience, and relentless devotion to family. My mom is the strongest person I know and simply the funniest. My "little" brother and sister have been my core their entire lives and introduced me to what it feels like to have your heart live outside of your body. And while my dad tried to warn him, Michael asked me anyway. Since then, we have trusted the process, grown into better versions of ourselves, and become damn good parents together.

Having all of you pour into Gabriel and into us has inspired this book and lifts us to do right by one another.

Do Right by Me

Introduction

The Gift

We are all one, and if we don't know it we will
learn it the hard way.

—**Bayard Rustin**,
organizer of the March on Washington, 1963

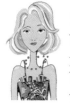 I wish I could say with certainty that this
book—and the passion, hope, and wisdom within its
pages—would have been birthed no matter how I
became a mother. However, one thing I can be sure of:
without my son, I may have never reckoned with the
story of the black experience in America. And I may not have
learned that my way of viewing things is not universal and not
always best, for my son or for me. Some of the prologue to my son's
arrival is relevant here.

On a gray and windy November day in 2000, I married Michael
D'Angelo, a handsome guy whom I met in college. Nearly all in
attendance at the suburban Philadelphia Catholic church that day
were, like us, white. All in all, a congregation comprised of pale
skin tones.

If this chapter were a film, you'd see time-lapse images of
leaves, snow, blooms, beach, pumpkins, snowmen, shamrocks, and
firecrackers all whizzing by, and then poof, before we knew it, we
had both endured and celebrated ten years of marriage. Sometimes I wonder how, and other days I revel in the wisdom of trust-
ing God and His process. There were plenty of times that I slipped

and got lazy, thinking, "It's in God's hands. There is nothing more for me to do," neglecting how essential I am in the process—my work, my diligence, my faith.

Marriage was marked by so many developments, changes, joy, pain, sunshine, rain. (If this chapter had a soundtrack, Rob Base and DJ EZ Rock's sampling of Frankie Beverly and Maze would be inserted here). One thing, however, nearly broke us and cemented us together: trying to have a baby.

It is very important here to note the intentional wording of "trying to have a baby" rather than what I have grown to demonize and loathe, the blanket phrase "starting a family." I don't mean to get overly sacramental here, but I felt sure that when Mike and I stood before hundreds of family and friends and said yes, we had started our family. We said yes to becoming one another's family, and we did it with witnesses!

What many didn't know, then and for many years afterward, was that Mike and I had been trying to get pregnant for nearly all ten years of our marriage. There were plenty of months and even years that we were not trying very vigorously, but in all that time, not a single pee stick was lit up with baby news. Even though I was unsure of myself in many aspects of being a wife and mother, I always had a deep longing to parent. I never really felt that I was cut out to be a wife, but I did think I could be a mom.

As Mike and I were toasting ten years of marriage, I was knee-deep in writing my dissertation proposal for my doctorate; we were both working full time in careers that were fulfilling and important to us; our mothers, siblings, and extended families were stable as ever; and I was finally starting to feel a rigid tension slip quietly away. After all these years of trying to have a baby, I was beginning to make peace with a possible future that our family would remain a family of two. In the spring of 2011, Mike was selected to join three faculty from his university to travel to Italy for a ten-day Franciscan pilgrimage. To add to this marvelous gift, spouses were invited to join; all Mike and I had to do was cover my costs. This ten-day pilgrimage not only promised to be a much-needed retreat for us but also provided time to contemplate growing our family.

Assisi and all of its magnificence could be chronicled in its own story. We savored the time, place, food, views, people, and reflection. By the time we returned home, we had decided to take the next steps that would lead to adopting a newborn. Those next steps included trees and trees of paperwork, background checks, soliciting support letters from friends, and sharing our decision with those closest to us. It culminated in an adoption class and home study with a social worker. The steps began early in June 2011, and we were declared "paper ready" to adopt by the second week in July. Every person with any shred of experience with the process of adoption repeated to us the very same caution: "Be patient. It could take a year or even two years. But it will happen." And every time I would remind myself, "Just breathe."

In August, I successfully (by the Grace of God) defended my doctoral dissertation proposal and felt confident that focusing on my research and final defense would be the perfect distraction from the anxiety of this looming wait. Mike's sister and sister-in-law gently probed for any opening to host a shower for us, but I swiftly expressed appreciation and declined their offer. With all the advice to be patient, I simply could not bear the thought of passing by a vacant nursery in our home. Our home remained without a stitch of Babies R Us to be found.

Over the summer months, our adoption facilitator had emailed us a couple birth mother profiles and asked us if we'd be interested in having her submit our profile to each birth mother's agency. Every time, we would say yes and try to contain the deliriousness of hope and fear. All the while, we enjoyed the end of summer and, both working at universities, prepared to ramp up for student orientations, move-in, and the start of the fall semester. The weekend was appropriately fun, and the return to the office was understandably sluggish. Mike and I got an email about a birth mother with a scheduled delivery that morning. We replied, "Of course, send our profile," and went about our day. A couple hours later, Mike called my cell phone, and I answered during a meeting in my office.

Me: "Hey! What's up?"
Mike: "We matched!"

The mix of incredulity, joy, and caution in his voice made his words indecipherable.

Me: "You called me at work to tell me that you matched your clothes today on your own?"
Mike: (lovingly) "Asshole. We matched! We have to get to South Carolina!"

Much like I wish we had hired a videographer for our wedding day, I wish that I had hired one to capture every detail of these minutes and all the minutes between Pennsylvania and South Carolina that followed. All we have is my recollection, which has been tinged by the sheer, voluminous waves of emotion that crashed over and into me from this very moment on. What I can tell you is there were many, many tears. No sleep. Gallons of coffee and water. More anxiety than my head and chest could hold. What I can tell you is that we called our moms and siblings, shed more tears, broke out a map (do we drive or fly?), figured out a plan to set up wire transfers with our bank in the morning, packed for a week (items that could be washed and worn however long we'd be gone), and plotted our course for South Carolina.

The next morning, we were in full motion. We each spoke with our bosses and had everyone's support to get our family-leave paperwork moving. We arrived at Mike's sister's house, where she and Mike's mom had spent all night washing, folding, and packing every stitch of our niece's baby clothes, as well as a bouncy seat, car seat, and portable crib to prepare our suddenly underequipped home. They threw in a case of diapers and wipes and offered shopping bags of fruit and snacks for the drive. More tears and a clear insistence for frequent calls and updates, with the promise of baby photos immediately upon our arrival at the hospital.

We got onto the turnpike at warp speed and headed to South Carolina, 670 miles away. I called my Aunt Jane to tell her our news and to confide that while I was bursting with excitement, there was this piercing question in my head: Because this baby had not grown inside of me, would either of us feel that sacred bond between mother and child? Without pause Jane said, "Kate, once they put that precious baby boy into your arms, it will happen." And with that, we were on our way.

It was 2:00 A.M. when we reached the exit for the hospital. Given the hour, and knowing from the adoption attorney's phone calls that the birth mother had been discharged and left the hospital before we arrived, we were thinking no one would expect us at the hospital. Mike and I looked into one another's puffy, bloodshot eyes and said, "Let's just try." I mean, who would think it strange that a babyless couple from Philadelphia showing up at a hospital in the middle of the night with a car filled with baby paraphernalia wouldn't have the very best of intentions?

We walked inside and were greeted by an elderly gentleman at the front desk before he contacted the nurse manager from the nursery to come meet us. Stunned by this hospitality, I thought for sure she was coming down to politely suggest we return during normal visiting hours. I prayed I could keep some composure. Mike and I nervously took the guest passes we were issued, and in minutes, a woman who embodied every bit of Southern hospitality glided toward us.

Looking back, I hope that we were capable of expressing gratitude or words, but I don't remember a thing other than how stunned I was by her warmth and generous embrace. My guess was that Mike and I found words and tossed them out there, hoping one or two would make sense. We stepped off the elevator, following obediently to what I thought would be a thick glass bank window where we could view the baby from a safe distance. The nurse pointed to the antibacterial dispenser next to the door, and we took our cue by lathering up as if preparing for surgery.

The dimly lit nursery had a soothing hum. A small band of pediatric nurses were speaking softly, checking charts, and monitoring machines and bassinets. I gracelessly lurched from side to side looking for The One. In fact, I was so busy rubbernecking that I missed the young nurse walking toward me and feeding a baby in her arms. Steps before colliding, she smiled and said, "You are just in time, mama. Your boy is ready for his bottle." And just as naturally as that, she slid Gabriel into my arms for the first time, and Aunt Jane's words echoed through my heart and soul. I turned to Mike, and no more words were needed. Our family of two became three.

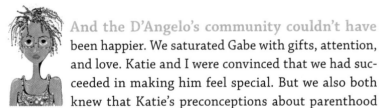 And the D'Angelo's community couldn't have been happier. We saturated Gabe with gifts, attention, and love. Katie and I were convinced that we had succeeded in making him feel special. But we also both knew that Katie's preconceptions about parenthood would have to expand to help her on the road she was on, one that she had not grown up expecting to be on. One of the many gifts that Gabriel, a beautiful biracial boy with one black and one white biological parent, brought to Katie and Mike's life has been to expand their experience of family and so much more.

Katie's view of what family looked like had been informed by a European or white American worldview. Societal messaging told her she needed to have a husband and biological child to have a real family. European American culture is generally more individualistic than African culture, focused primarily on a nuclear family that includes parents and siblings. The reality that a biological child might not be forthcoming was particularly painful for Katie.

Like Katie, I was married and was never pregnant. Unlike Katie, I am black and am most informed by an African worldview. I am certainly not suggesting that black women do not experience disappointment and pain at the reality of not having biological children. They do. However, an African worldview provides a perspective on family that is expansive and communal. Not having a husband or biological children does not mean not having family.

While there is no universal African American family system or European American model, and no one can say that all black families look the same or all white families look the same, there are common threads that emanate from an African philosophical value system that we see in many black families. Similarly, there are some common behaviors that we see in white families. For example, African Americans and Africans throughout the diaspora generally view the concept of family more broadly than European or white Americans. The core family includes not only parents and siblings but also grandparents, aunts, uncles, and cousins, all of whom may live in the same household or in nearby communities. Persons of similar age who have close relational ties often refer to each other as cousins even if there is no biological connection. And young persons who grow up in the same household with others in their age group may think of each other as siblings and refer to each other as brother or sister, although they may be biologically cousins or have no biological relationship at all. Biology is simply less important than relationship. In this same vein, African Americans commonly view familial responsibilities as going beyond the nuclear family. Notably, in traditional African cultures, there was no concept of the nuclear family; rather, the community formed the basis for the family unit and the notion of standing in the gap for others, even in a parenting role, was familiar and without shame. This perspective allows one to see boundless opportunities to nurture children regardless of biological ties. You can be good to children, love and support them, and contribute to their development in ways that are meaningful and have eternal impact.

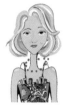 I was operating within a different cultural paradigm. One that imposed upon its participants a notion that you are only good enough and have enough if you measure up to a predetermined set of standards, in this case a heterosexual marriage and biological babies. And one that judged others as inferior in order to feel superior.

Gabe helped me see more clearly that the worldview and value system that I feel most at home in is neither the only one available nor the best. The mindset that I'd inherited certainly wasn't doing me any good, and my ability to shift gears brought me the greatest gift of my life. Gabe expanded my horizons, and by learning to support him and give him the cultural tools he will need as a black man in America not only helps him but also helps me. Other value systems are different, not deficient. Each is a unique and equally valid reflection of humanity. Gabe showed me that the family I had all along was always so much more than just Mike and me. I realized that we have a vast and wonderful family, some but not all with whom we share biological ties. Once I could see, I felt freed from pain that had long blocked my view, and it opened me up to the incredible abundance of family and community that would grow into ours.

Katie and I decided to tell our story and share our conversation in this book with the hope that it informs and supports people raising black children in white families, communities, and other spaces.

We began the book with adoptive parents and adopted children in mind. Around 140,000 children are adopted by families in the United States each year; nearly 100 million Americans have adoption in their immediate family, whether this includes adopting, placing, or being adopted; and there are about 1.5 million adopted children in the United States, which is 2 percent of the population. The Institute on Family Studies found that substantial numbers of Asian, Hispanic, multiracial, and black adoptees in the United States were being raised by parents of a different race or ethnicity than themselves. That includes 90 percent of Asian adoptees, 64 percent of multiracial adoptees, 62 percent of Hispanic adoptees, and 55 percent of black adoptees. Overall, 44 percent of adopted kindergarten students were being cared for by adoptive parents of a different race or ethnicity. By contrast, only 3 percent of white adoptees had been adopted by a mother of a different race or ethnicity. We will start where we began: with a conversation about transracial adoption.

1

Knowing What You Don't Know

Not to know is bad;
not to wish to know is worse.

—**African proverb**

Although the black community tends to be pretty accepting, some black people are reluctant to accept white families parenting black children. An experience with Gabe reminded me of that.

I babysat while Katie and Mike had a date night. I secured Gabe in his stroller, and we took off for a walk around the D'Angelos' neighborhood. As we passed the YMCA, a woman I went to high school with and hadn't seen in probably three decades spotted us and said, "Val Harrison?" I recognized her immediately, and we greeted each other with a hug and smile. Gabe was nine months old, and I was forty-nine years old. The woman acknowledged that Gabe was the cutest baby ever but chuckled and said, "Girrrrrl! You waited this long to have a baby?"

"Oh no," I assured her, "I'm Aunt Val." We laughed and ended a short but pleasant encounter.

I couldn't help but think that my schoolmate's response to Katie may have been different. Katie may be confronted by people who are opposed to transracial adoption. I wanted to help her understand where the pushback, side-eyes, and challenges that might be hurled at her over the years come from. I also wondered how she would handle herself if confronted, so I converted one of our pleasant but predictable office conversations into an inquisition. I retreated from my initial inclination to fire questions and instead tossed them gently. I wanted her to be able to handle herself, to take and defend a position, or to mention a study or two. But she didn't. She retreated.

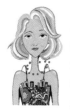 I understand why Val wanted me to be able to respond to the statement that white parents cannot raise black children. And not just to respond, but to answer poised and confidently while being astutely grounded in the research. However, I wasn't ready then. Now, because I know this moment will come, I am certain in my response, yet I'm only beginning to learn all that I need to know.

"You can't know what you don't know." That's how Beth Hall, transracial adoptive parent and director of PACT, An Adoption Alliance, summarized the quandary in which many white adoptive parents of black children find themselves. Very thorough and important research has been done on transracial adoption, and we are grateful for those who dove in to study the subject and reemerged with perspectives and information that have added to the discussion. This book is our effort to make some of that research more accessible to you. We firmly believe that knowledge of an issue is the first step in conquering its challenges.

Let's set a few parameters before we get started. First, this book is not intended to be an exhaustive examination of the research on transracial adoption. Rather, we want to provide parents with an orientation to how race will impact their child's life, informed by research and our lived experiences, so that they are equipped to raise healthy, confident, and well-adjusted children. Second, this work focuses primarily on the adoption by white families of black children. We have defined a black child as a child with at least one biological parent who is of African descent, and here's why. Most often a child having at least one biological parent of African descent will have observable characteristics such as skin color, hair texture, or other physical features that differ in varying degrees from their white adoptive parents. Notably, if a child has any visible characteristics associated with people of African descent, it is likely that he or she will be regarded by others as black.

Our use of the nomenclature *black* is not indicative of any commentary or disregard of other terms such as *persons of color, biracial, interracial, African American*, or *brown*. What drives us is a concern that regardless of the chosen nomenclature, children regarded by others as black need to be equipped with positive racial identity and other strategies to navigate the complexities and burden of that identification in the United States. The focus of this book is on race, but there may be other factors such as disability, gender, ethnicity, or sexuality that intersect with and must be navigated along with race. Finally, while the initial impetus for this book was to support transracial adoptive families, we believe the book can be helpful for other communities raising black children, including black or interracial families of origin.

If you are reading this book, you probably have at least heard the term *transracial adoption*, or TRA. It is the term used most often to describe the adoption of a child "when the child's race/ethnicity is different from that of both parents."[1] According to a 2008 Evan B. Donaldson Adoption Institute report, "throughout most of the 19th century and beyond, transracial adoption in the United States rarely occurred and, as a result of racism institutionalized in law, it was illegal in many states."[2]

The origins of transracial adoption in the United States can be traced back to times of war. World War II, as well as subsequent wars in Korea and Vietnam, tore apart families in those countries and left many children parentless. In the 1950s, Japanese, Korean, and Vietnamese children were among the first children of color adopted by white American parents. International adoptions were soon followed by adoption of Native American and black children by white American families.[3]

Transracial adoption involving black children and white families gained momentum in the 1960s, some believe fueled by (1) a civil rights movement that "altered societal views of racial relationships" toward notions of integration and (2) declining numbers of white children available for adoption "as a result of changing attitudes about single parenting, the legalization of abortion, and the increased use of contraceptives."[4] A 1987 study estimates more than 2,500 transracial adoptions involving black children by 1971. Many people met these adoptions with skepticism and resistance.[5]

For example, in 1972, the National Association of Black Social Workers (NABSW) published a position paper on transracial adoption of black children by white families, opposing the practice of screening out potential black adoptive families in favor of white families. Rather, NABSW advocated for black children remaining in black families "in order that they receive the total sense of themselves and develop a sound projection of their future."[6] NABSW's chief concern was that white families might lack the resources and knowledge to equip a black child to develop positive racial identity and navigate life in a racist society.[7] The NABSW position paper explained:

> The family is the basic unit of society; one's first, most pervasive and only consistent culturing life experience. Humans develop their sense of values, identity, self-concept, attitudes and basic perspective within the family group. Black children in white homes are cut off from the healthy development of themselves as black people, which development is the normal expectation and only true humanistic goal.[8]

NABSW cited three particular areas of concern. First, the paper noted the importance of family resemblance to positive identity and expressed a concern that the process of developing positive racial identity could be frustrated when a black child does not resemble any relative. Second, the position statement assumed that white parents would be unable to teach black children about the realities the black child was soon to experience. Finally, they argued that black children in white homes would not be taught coping techniques to deal with racism.[9]

Researchers attribute a swift decline in the number of transracial adoptions in the early 1970s to the NABSW position paper.[10] However, the larger number of black children in temporary foster care than available black adoptive families—despite the willingness and readiness of these families to adopt—spawned a resurgence in transracial adoption in the succeeding decades.[11]

Scholars have disagreed on the efficacy of transracial adoption. Much of the early research found transracial adoption is both safe and preferable to institutional care. Generally, these studies found that children adopted transracially in the United States or from other countries had overall adjustment outcomes similar to children placed in same-race families.[12] The 2008 Donaldson report was somewhat equivocal about this first wave of research because it perceived the work as being more limited in scope and less rigorous in terms of methodology than later scholarship.[13]

Subsequent researchers were careful not to overlook some of the challenges of transracial adoption, including black children struggling with feeling different, accepted, and comfortable with their physical appearance, particularly those living in all-white communities.[14] Similarly, studies found that transracially adopted children often struggle to develop a positive racial/ethnic identity.[15] The Donaldson report tracked the research over the next several decades and found that the weight of authority agreed that "transracial adoption in itself does not produce psychological or social maladjustment problems in children" and that "transracially adopted children and their families face a range of challenges, and the manner in which parents handle them facilitates or hinders children's development."[16] Specifically, the research found "when parents facilitate their children's understanding of and comfort with their own ethnicities, the children show more positive adjustment in terms of higher levels of self-esteem, lower feelings of marginality, greater ethnic pride, less distress, and better psychological adjustment."[17] Similarly, when black teenagers have been socialized to be conscious of and able to respond to racism, researchers have found that they have higher self-esteem and personal efficacy.[18] Still another group of researchers weighed in with their belief that any negative impact with respect to identity is outweighed by the benefits of transracial adoption.[19]

In a 1994 restatement of its 1972 position paper, NABSW continued to advocate for same-race adoption as optimal for black children but appeared somewhat more sympathetic to transracial adoption in order to place more children who needed homes.[20] Federal legislation followed public opinion in support of transracial adoption by generally prohibiting adoption agencies from considering race in adoption placements and requiring that state agencies make diligent efforts to recruit foster and adoptive parents who represent the racial and ethnic backgrounds of children in foster care.[21]

Beth Hall of PACT also stresses the significance of the perspectives and voices of black adult transracial adoptees who are now writing and sharing their journeys and instructing us on how to improve experiences for black children in white families. Chad Goller-Sojourner is an African American adult transracial adoptee, educator, coach, writer, performer, and author.[22] In 1972, when he was thirteen months old, he was adopted by white parents and raised in a white suburb of Tacoma, Washington. Despite his parents' every effort to seek out diverse schools, infuse their home with books by black authors, and expose their children to people of all races, Goller-Sojourner is clear: there was a limit to what his parents could provide.[23] Through his extensive work and various creative mediums, Goller-Sojourner confirms what the research tells us. Families must intentionally enable a healthy racial identity. For too many years, Goller-Sojourner explains, his "truth resulted in a long, lonely, and painful journey to a healthy racial identity. While my parents did the best they could with what they knew, like me, they didn't know much. We had no benefit of history or hindsight, institutional support, books to guide us, or even ways of knowing what we were getting right or wrong. Instead we found ourselves being the clinical trials and day laborers of a grand and complex social experiment known as transracial adoption."[24]

Self-described multicultural educator, transracial adoptee, adoptive parent, and scholar activist John Raible was one of the "angry adoptees" in the 1998 training film *Struggle for Identity: Issues in Transracial Adoption*.[25] Much of his research and teaching has been motivated and inspired not only by his own experience as a transracial adoptee but also as an adoptive parent of two young men. Raible has published a substantial body of research on the subject of identity and transracial adoption.[26] As an educator, Raible shows a keen awareness of the parent and child relationship, and his work explores the transracial adolescent in the classroom and the critical role of the teacher in setting the principles for the learning environment.

Here's what we know. Black children do best when they have positive racial identity or when they feel good about being a member of their racial or ethnic group. Their achievement and well-being depend on it. Conversely, confusion about racial/ethnic identity is linked to behavior problems and psychological distress. The well-being of black children is also tied to their ability to deal with racism.[27] Thus, a key takeaway is the undeniable need to help black children develop positive racial identity and equip them with the necessary life skills to navigate the racism that is entrenched in American society. This book can serve to show

parents why these skills are necessary and how to go about cultivating them.

Neither positive black identity nor life skills to navigate racism
can be achieved without learning the race narrative of the United
States and how racist systems continue to impact the lives of black
and white people today.

2

Trapped in History

Until the story of the hunt is told by the lion, the
tale of the hunt will always glorify the hunter.

—AFRICAN PROVERB

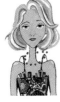 James Baldwin's words "trapped in history" are
a constant reminder that outcomes in any given situa-
tion may turn on race. It was the end of a very long
week of work, and I was eking along my always traf-
ficked road home during peak rush hour. The city makes
up 8.5 miles of my 9-mile commute, and there is never a quick way
to get through it. Some drivers treat it like *Frogger* and attempt to
weave in and out of two packed lanes. My patience tends to wear
thin by mile two.

It's dark by 5 P.M. because it was January, and it was also cold
and dreary. As I pushed on my brakes after coasting my next car-
length forward, a slightly larger SUV attempting to move from
behind me misjudged the space and crunched my left rear bumper.
I hoped it would be an insignificant tap to my thirteen-year-old
hybrid. The other car's passenger rolled down his window, and out
gazed the face of a twentysomething brown-skinned boy with a
hoodie around his head who coolly determined for me, "It's good.
It's good. There's nothing there."

Oh, how I want to believe him. As I opened my door to get out and look, I could hear what the endless sea of drivers behind us must be thinking: "Please just get out of my way."

I inspected the bumper, and it was cracked like an old Frisbee. My eyes returned to the car's passenger, and I said, "Nope. It's actually not good at all."

By now the driver had gotten out of his car and walked around to see what he'd missed. This modestly dressed man was also twentysomething, and he also had a skin shade of brown. He was visibly shaken. I asked him if he was okay and if he'd be comfortable driving into the parking lot across the street to exchange info and get out of the traffic. He agreed. I said in my sweetest, most nonthreatening white lady voice, "I'm just going to take a picture of your license plate first."

As we were waiting for the light to turn, his vehicle behind mine, my brain raced through a checklist of what to do in the event of an accident. Driver's license. Registration. Insurance card and contact info. Hopefully we didn't have to call the police because the last time I was in a car accident in the city at rush hour, we waited forty minutes, and they never showed.

We pulled into the empty lot, and all three of us exited our vehicles and returned to the busted corner of my car. The hazy, cool passenger, looking at the damage he'd denied, said, "Nah, man. You didn't do that. You touched this back part. That part wasn't you."

Now I was annoyed. Nice white lady was about to exit and hand off the baton to the not-nice one. But the driver quickly interceded. "Stop. This was my fault. I heard that big truck hit his horn and got nervous. I'm really sorry."

A white guy in a Suburban pulled up, looked at me, and asked, "Everything okay?"

I responded first. "Yup, just a fender bender. We're good, thanks."

The driver and I returned to our exchange, and his passenger proceeded to either make or take a call. He very quickly realized that he didn't have his insurance information or his license on him. He did produce his registration, which I took a phone photo of and silently prayed that it was his name and home address. I asked him if I could hold it to take the picture because his hands were shaking so much that I couldn't get it to focus. He also produced his college parking permit hangtag. This evidence came with the words, "I'm a college student and am home for the weekend."

I took his number and called him while we stood there under the street lamp so he would have my number too. Okay—I also did it that way to be sure he gave me his real number. Arguably, I had enough data that if he was really playing to my heart, I could call a police friend and track him down.

I told him we could speak later by phone and asked him to send me a photo of his insurance information when he found it. We agreed and got in our cars, and I resumed my path home.

When I got home and worked my way through the details with Mike, he winced when I mentioned that I did not get his insurance info. However, he quickly moved ahead and said, "I am very proud of you for not calling the police."

That stung a little, partly because it felt like an accusation and partly because these days, our awareness of the ways race could turn an encounter scared us now. Since we'd adopted Gabe seven years earlier, I became more tuned in to the reality that police may not offer a feeling of comfort or security in this situation, particularly for persons of color, and I was not used to it. My instinct was not to contact the police when that accident occurred because all I wanted to do was get home, and waiting on the police would have prolonged me getting there. It wasn't that I feared for these two young men if the cops showed up to this scene. Rather, I did not wish to be further inconvenienced.

Mike likely should have picked another word instead of *proud*. It wasn't so much pride as it was agreement that I'd chosen wisely in the moment. What I could not have known when I was actively choosing not to call the police was how the whole thing would have gone south when the driver didn't have the proper documents and discovered what we all did the next morning: that the driver was not insured. Had my discomfort with the situation led me to bring police to the scene, they would doubtless have made this a more costly mistake for the driver—a risk I wonder whether I would have been as ready to run if the other driver had been a white woman.

The driver texted me later that night, and we exchanged more texts the next day. His texts included several rounds of "I really am sorry." But then came, "My aunt dropped me from her policy a few months ago and I didn't know. I understand that it is illegal to drive without insurance. I understand that you have to do what you have to do."

Of course I couldn't wait to process this whole thing with Val.

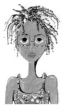 In *Dreams from My Father*, President Barack Obama tells a story about his grandmother's encounter with a black man who asked her for money as she waited for a bus. After the exchange with the man, who showed no evidence that he was a threat of danger, President Obama's grandmother was afraid to take the bus to work the next day and insisted that her husband drive her. The story revealed the struggle of many persons who are well meaning but underinformed about issues of race and racism in America. President Obama recalls:

> I sat on the edge of my bed and thought about my grandparents. They had sacrificed again and again for me. They had poured all their lingering hopes into my success. Never had they given me reason to doubt their love; I doubted if they ever would. And yet I knew that men who might easily have been my brothers could still inspire their rawest fears.[1]

Katie wasn't afraid of the young men simply because they were black, because they wore hoodies, because they were young, because they didn't have an insurance card, or any combination of the above. She had struggled with what informs irrational fears, and her evolving perspective was evident. She recognizes that outcomes for the young black college students could be much different from the outcomes for two young white men in the same situation, regardless of a young white man's background or educational level; more on that in Chapter 7. This is certainly not to suggest that police intervention is never appropriate, but Katie, Mike, and I, and many others, feel compelled to engage in a process that assesses the risk to them versus whatever benefit we would derive from police involvement in a minor fender bender. In the rest of this chapter, we explain the compulsion by examining where the stigma that shapes how black people are viewed comes from historically.

When many white individuals meet or exceed social landmarks of achievement, they often relish the myth that their success is solely the fruit of their labor and not because of a larger system designed to benefit them (and harm others) centuries before they were born. Some will not accept the premise that we all need to look back and understand the impact of systems of privilege and disadvantage today. Moreover, some white people who have faced adversity and struggle tend to be even less tolerant, their awareness of the particular disadvantage that they've overcome leading them to ignore how a different skin color would have made their journey even more difficult because of racism. You can find many definitions of the term *racism*, but generally, it refers to a "system of structuring opportunity and assigning value based on the social interpretation of how one looks (which is what we call 'race') that unfairly disadvantages some individuals and communities, unfairly advantages other individuals and communities, and saps the strength of the whole society through the waste of human resources."[2] Understanding the system is a necessary first step toward achieving racial equity.

Undergirding this system is the doctrine of white racial supremacy. There are concepts (like white racial supremacy) and other topics, words, and notions that are being offered in this book that may make you feel uncomfortable. Arguably, there will be people who feel we didn't push the discomfort level enough. Wherever you find yourself, this chapter intends to walk you through centuries of our shared history. Chances are this is not how you heard or read your history in school. Nonetheless, we believe that having a more accurate foundation is essential to discerning the influence of race on this country's laws, policies, and practices. One of the tools that we have found helpful when teaching this subject in the classroom is an engaging activity borrowed from board games like *Life* that we call *The Walk*. It requires participants to gain and lose ground as they move with the history that describes how racism took root in this country. As the instructor traces historical events that affect the relative status of black and white Americans, they invite students to step forward and backward to mark the relative distance to cover to reach equality and the persistance of the innovations and developments pushing them apart. It also reinforces that history is not always progressive, starting from a supposed backward state and slowly becoming reformed. While participants in the physical exercise have the advantage of seeing the gap continue to widen visually, readers of this book have the advantage of being able to see the whole historic record on the page in front of them at once and review each development at their pace.

Although laws in their various forms have been used as an instrument of subjugation of Africans in the United States since shortly after their arrival on the shores of Jamestown, Virginia, in 1619, the story of black people did not begin there. Significant African history takes us back to 2500 B.C., when black Africans finished building the pyramids. However, four hundred years of European slave trade and colonization have distorted the popular impressions of African history and culture that we have inherited.

White racial supremacy uses skin color as a barometer of worth. According to the doctrine, paleness equals superiority. This construction has led to an effort on the part of some white people to dominate all over the world and attributes performance and behavior to racial differences in order to justify slavery, oppression, terrorism, and differential treatment. Europeans justified subjugation through colonialism by claiming it was as an act of charity, a generous uplift of societies they were convinced were less because they were different and darker, a moral responsibility they called "the white man's burden." In the seventeenth century, Africans were involuntarily brought by Europeans to the United States as part of the European slave trade. African and African American history scholar Molefi K. Asante describes the horror of the journey:

> The ancestors of the present African Americans were stolen from the continent of Africa, placed on ships against their wills, and transported across the Atlantic. While most of the enslaved Africans went to Brazil and Cuba, a great portion landed in the Southern States of the United States. At the height of the European Slave Trade almost every nation in Europe was involved in some aspect of the enterprise. As the "trade" grew more profitable and the European captains became more ambitious, larger ships with specially built "slave galleries" were commissioned. These galleries between the decks were no more than eighteen inches in height. Needless to say, many Africans perished under such conditions. The North made the shipping of Africans its business; the South made the working of Africans its business. By 1860, the Census counted four and a half million Africans in the United States.[3]

Thus, black people start their journey in America at the extreme disadvantage of having arrived not only against their volition but also as expendable cargo, commodities of a system made to profit from their violation and content to harm and kill them in bulk for the sake of efficiency. The year 1860 marked the secession of the American South, and by this point, while most enslaved Africans were held on Southern plantations, the North enjoyed the fruits of an American economy subsidized by captive labor.

In 1619 in Virginia, there was no law referencing the status of black people. A white individual manning the ship that carried the first Africans to Jamestown is referred to in Virginia records not as a white man but as a "Dutchman."[4] While there is some disagreement among historians, most take the position that the enslavement of Africans did not begin in the United States until 1660, and prior to that time, white and black laborers in Virginia held virtually the same position.[5]

The first slave code dates back to 1680 Virginia and served as a "model of repression throughout the South for the next 180 years."[6] It read:

> Whereas the frequent meetings of considerable numbers of Negro slaves under pretense of feasts and burials is judged of dangerous consequences [be it] enacted that no Negro or slave may carry arms, such as any club, staff, gun, sword, or other weapon, nor go from his owner's plantation without a certificate and then only on necessary occasions; the punishment twenty lashes on the bare back, well laid on. And further, if any Negro lift up his hand against any Christian he shall receive thirty lashes, and if he absent himself or lie out from his master's service and resist lawful apprehension, he may be killed and this law shall be published every six months.[7]

Although science has established that there is only one biological race and humans are genetically virtually 100 percent the same, America nonetheless created a story that attributed significance to skin color.

By the Revolutionary era, race was widely used, and its meaning had solidified as a reference for social categories of Indians, blacks, and whites [citations omitted]. More than that, race signified a new ideology about human differences and a new way of structuring society that had not existed before in human history. *The fabrication of a new type of categorization for humanity was needed because the leaders of the American colonies at the turn of the 18th century had deliberately selected Africans to be permanent slaves. In an era when the dominant political philosophy was equality, civil rights, democracy, justice, and freedom for all human beings, the only way Christians could justify slavery was to demote Africans to nonhuman status* [emphasis added]. The humanity of the Africans was debated throughout the 19th century, with many holding the view that Africans were created separately from other, more human, beings.[8]

And so began the codification of black subjugation and white privilege in the United States, which included physical and mental trauma resulting from intentionally tearing apart black families and stripping them of their language, history, and culture; inhumane working conditons; and the rape, brutal beatings, disfigurement, and murder of black people at the hands of white people. In the words of author James Baldwin, one of the most compelling voices to tell the story of the black experience in the United States, "black people were told that they weren't worth shit and everything around them confirmed it."[9]

The onslaught that followed included the ratification of the U.S. Constitution in 1787, which addressed the issue of race in like manner. The highest law of the land considered Africans to be three-fifths of a person for purposes of apportioning representation.[10] But no one was representing them anyway—they weren't allowed to vote, and no one in power considered them a constituency. Had the Constitution counted them as full people for purposes of apportionment, that would have increased, not decreased, the power of Southern slaveholders in the federal government. No mistake, the Constitution preserved slavery with Article IV Section 2, stating that "no Person held to Service or Labour in one State, under the Laws thereof, escaping into another, shall, in Consequence of any Law or Regulation therein, be discharged from such Service or Labour, but shall be delivered up on Claim of the Party to whom such Service or Labour may be due," giving those who enslaved Africans a constitutional right to retrieve them even if the state they escaped to did not recognize slavery.[11] The three-fifths definition of enslaved personhood was negotiated by the white North to moderate the power of the white South. All of which is to say the Constitutional debate treated black people as pawns in someone else's political game, not as citizens of the republic being formed. The Consitution also gave specific permission to continue the international slave trade.[12]

During this same period, the concept of a free public school system was also being formed. Many states share the same model of school organization and funding, so we will use our home state, Pennsylvania, as the exemplar.[13] In 1854, Pennsylvania's lawmakers were at work putting substance on the framework for a free public education system. Although the Gradual Abolition Act of 1780[14] abolished slavery in Pennsylvania, the law made it clear that black children should not be afforded the same educational opportunities as their white counterparts.

The directors or controllers of the several districts of the state, are hereby authorized and required to establish within their respective districts, *separate schools for the tuition of negro and mulatto children* [emphasis added], whenever such schools can be so located as to accommodate twenty or more pupils; and whenever such separate schools shall be established, and kept open four months in any year, the directors or controllers *shall not be compelled to admit such pupils into any other schools of the district* [emphasis added]: Provided, that in cities or boroughs, the board of controllers shall provide for such schools out of the general funds assessed and collected by uniform taxation for educational purposes.[15]

As schools were equipping children to take advantage of an economy that would favor an educated workforce, lawmakers ensured that black children would never receive the same quality education as white children to take advantage of emerging opportunities. Lawmakers reinforced the scheme by manipulating the flow of money. This same year, the first funding formula for public education was designed. Pennsylvania's lawmakers at the 1873 Constitutional Convention considered a uniform system of funding—meaning they would spend the same amount educating each child in the commonwealth—but specifically rejected the inclusion of the word *uniform* so that local districts could use their own resources to add to the resources provided by the state, even if this system resulted in vastly different educational experiences for children in school districts throughout the commonwealth.[16] Thus, the system was designed to be unequal. The original intent and design of the present funding scheme was to have local communities provide children with the best education that the particular community could afford. Almost a decade later in 1881, the Pennsylvania legislature reversed its previous stance on segregation in education and made it unlawful for school administrators and teachers to require black children to go to separate schools.[17] However, the funding scheme was virtually unchanged. Thus, schools in wealthy communities, of which previously enslaved black people were rarely a part, had the most resourced schools, while fewer financial resources went to schools in the poorest communities, in which black people were disproportionately overrepresented.

In most U.S. states today, public educational services are funded through a combination of federal, state, and local resources but still rely most heavily on local community resources. On average, federal funds make up only 8 percent of the resources provided for K–12 public education.[18] In our hometown of Philadelphia, for example, the local resources, which represent more than 50 percent of the funds dedicated to K–12 public education, are collected primarily through property taxes. The contribution from the state to fund K–12 schools in Pennsylvania hovers around 34 percent of the school district budget.[19] Thus, on top of the inequalities introduced by the slave trade and the legal frameworks of early America, the American schooling system introduces new disadvantages to black Americans.

In like manner, the mid-nineteenth-century U.S. Supreme Court confirmed its commitment to white hegemony in the 1857 *Dred Scott* case.[20] The question before the Supreme Court was whether an African, whose ancestors were involuntarily brought to the United States and sold into slavery, could become a citizen of the United States within the meaning of the Constitution. The court decided that "neither the class of persons who had been imported as slaves, nor their descendants, whether they had become free or not, were then acknowledged as part of the people, nor intended to be included in the general words used in that memorable instrument."[21] In reaching this decision, a majority of the justices concluded:

> [The black race] had for more than a century before been regarded as beings of an inferior order, and altogether unfit to associate with the white race, either in social or political relations; and so far inferior, that they had no rights which the white man was bound to respect; and that the Negro might justly and lawfully be reduced to slavery for his benefit.[22]

Although the country's Declaration of Independence proclaimed, "We hold these truths to be self-evident: that all men are created equal,"[23] the *Dred Scott* court concluded that black persons

could not have been among the "all men" who were "created equal";
otherwise, they reasoned, white men would be acting in a manner
utterly inconsistent with their words by enslaving and denying
them basic human rights.[24] The *Dred Scott* case formalized how far
the status of black people had been lowered so that the country
could justify slavery. It took all protection under the law from
black people in America, enslaved or free.

In 1863, President Abraham Lincoln issued the Emancipation
Proclamation, which declared, "All persons held as slaves within
any state or designated part of a state, the people whereof shall
then be in rebellion against the United States, shall be then,
thenceforward, and forever, free."[25] Slavery was for the most part
constitutionally abolished in December 1865 by the Thirteenth
Amendment:

> Neither slavery nor involuntary servitude, except as a pun-
> ishment for crime whereof the party shall have been duly
> convicted, shall exist within the United States, or any place
> subject to their jurisdiction.[26]

The Thirteenth Amendment, along with the 1868 Citizenship
Clause of the Fourteenth Amendment,[27] which provided that "all
persons born or naturalized in the United States, and subject to
the jurisdiction thereof, are citizens of the United States and of
the State wherein they reside" effectively overturned *Dred Scott*.

What followed was a Reconstruction period, which ran through
1877 and provided some relief for formerly enslaved Africans in
the form of access to Congress and constitutional amendments
and federal laws reinforcing the citizenship of black people and
their protection under the law.[28] In 1870 and 1875, Mississippi's
Hiram Revels and Blanche Bruce, respectively, became the first
two African American senators.

However, the gains of the Reconstruction era were short-lived
and the last progress toward equality for some time, due in part to

the activity of white terrorist organizations, racial segregation or "Jim Crow" laws, and Supreme Court rulings hostile to the interests of African Americans.[29] The United States would not see its third African American senator for nearly one hundred years when, in 1967, the citizens of Massachusetts elected Edward Brooke. While the Thirteenth Amendment mandated that citizenship could not be stripped on the basis of race, new laws sprung up that restricted the vote to citizens who had already voted before, or who were vouched for by persons who'd voted before, or on the basis of a fee or a test meant to screen out black voters who lacked the resources of existing white voters. And those are only the legal obstacles placed on voting; there was also the practical matter of state-sanctioned violence against black people brave enough to try to exercise their rights of citizenship.

In 1896, the U.S. Supreme Court again had the opportunity to expand or limit the rights of black people in the *Plessy v. Ferguson* case.[30] The issue in the case was whether the state of Louisiana could require black people and white people to ride in separate railway cars. However, what was at stake in this ruling was so much more than railway cars. The decision would be used to justify separate schools and other public spaces. The Supreme Court approved the concept that separate public facilities of equal quality were in fact legal. In its strained analysis, the court exposed its fear that "if . . . the colored race should become the dominant power in the state legislature, and should enact a law in precisely similar terms, it would thereby relegate the white race to an inferior position."[31] The Supreme Court's language confirmed that the abolition of slavery had not erased the hegemonic viewpoint under which that system thrived.

Despite laws prohibiting white terrorist activities, in the first fourteen years of the twentieth century, there were more than 1,100 black people lynched, most in the Southern states but in Northern states as well.[32] Lynching created a consistent danger but also enforced a state of fear among black people that to live their lives with the full dignity of their white neighbors would invite the retribution of the mob. Lynching was not punished by the state, and indeed, white communities treated it as an entertaining event at which to see and be seen. The culture of Jim Crow's America reasserted the control and special status of white people that had previously been enforced through slavery.

During the first several decades of the twentieth century, the United States was on an economic high. Industry was booming, and around 1916, Southern blacks began migrating north to take advantage of the promise of economic opportunities. They would not find the same opportunities as their white neighbors, but they could find jobs.

Then the stock market crash of October 1929 threw the United States into what is known as the Great Depression. Afraid and anxious, consumers spent less and investors invested less. As a result, companies were forced to lay off workers as the demand for products and services plummeted. At its worst, the toll of the unemployed exceeded fifteen million Americans.[33]

The Great Depression revealed significant structural problems that President Franklin D. Roosevelt, who took office in 1933, quickly worked to address. The relief efforts were known as the New Deal. Ira Katznelson traces significant events following the Great Depression and concludes that many of the New Deal programs that appeared to be race neutral were intentionally discriminatory in favor of white people in order to perpetuate white privilege while at the same time blocking black people from participating in this economic revival.[34] For example, the New Deal legislation created unions, set minimum required wages, regulated the number of hours that employees could be forced to work, and established Social Security, all for the purpose of helping Americans regain financial stability and build a middle class. At the same time, black people were overrepresented in jobs as farmworkers and maids. These groups—constituting more than 60 percent of the black labor force and nearly 75 percent of those who were employed in the South—were initially excluded from these wealth- and life-enhancing pieces of legislation. Consequently, writes Katznelson, "at the very moment when a wide array of public policies was providing most white Americans with valuable tools to advance their social welfare—insure their old age through social security, get good jobs, acquire economic security, build assets, and gain middle-class status—most black Americans were left behind or left out. Affirmative action then was white."[35]

Federal home ownership policies provided yet another vehicle to further push white families forward economically while holding black families back. Shortly before the New Deal, a typical mortgage required a large down payment and full repayment within about ten years. At the urging of President Roosevelt, Congress created the Home Owners' Loan Corporation (HOLC) in 1933 and then the Federal Housing Administration (FHA) in 1934. HOLC offered federal bonds to lenders in exchange for mortgages already in default, providing new fifteen-year mortgages at 5 percent interest to homeowners, allowing easier repayment on their debt to the government. The FHA-insured private mortgages resulted in a drop in interest rates and a smaller down payment required to buy a house. Banks could offer loans requiring no more than 10 percent down that could be paid over twenty to thirty years because FHA insured the loans. This FHA mandate to insure privately held home mortgages was a way to bolster the housing market during the Depression. However, the FHA refused to invest in racially mixed neighborhoods, channeling most of its funding to predominantly white areas, allowing white families to acquire an intergenerational asset that would serve as a nest egg for their children and create a wealth gap that persists to this day, and making sure America's healthy and depressed neighborhoods remained determined by race.

FHA strengthened its practice of refusing to insure loans, or insuring loans on less favorable terms, in certain urban neighborhoods through the use of maps developed by HOLC. Any neighborhood deliberately excluded was identified in red.[36] Most often, the racial composition of the neighborhood determined the amount of FHA investment. In addition, the FHA manual instructed evaluators to rate mortgage risks based on potential changes in the racial and class composition of the community. In addition, those properties that had restrictive covenants connected to them—or specific contractual provisions that prevented sale of the property to black persons—received the greatest investment.[37]

After 1949, the government could no longer legally continue its practice of housing exclusion because of the passage of the Housing Act of 1949. However, in activity known as blockbusting, real estate agents heavily solicited white homeowners, sold or bought for themselves houses from fleeing white residents at reduced prices, and quickly sold or rented them at inflated prices to incoming black residents.[38]

By the mid-1950s, the FHA and Veterans Administration investment greatly aided urban home buyers of all races in purchasing an affordable first home. But black people were locked out of developing suburbs like Levittown, Pennsylvania. Levittown is just outside of Philadelphia, and William Levitt was one of the first and largest producers of suburban housing characterized by single family homes with lawns, garages, driveways, and increasing property values. And with property appreciation came further wealth-building for white families. Redlining was outlawed by now, but the federal government refused to subsidize developers who sold to black families. As a result, these communities were generally off limits to black families, and they were denied the same opportunity to build intergenerational wealth.[39]

The Philadelphia Commission on Human Relations performed a revealing test in the mid-1960s. Black and white field representatives visited real estate offices asking for information about available houses in the same area. The list shown to the white testers differed from that shown to black people, proving that agents were still driving segregation. During an investigation into unethical soliciting, one of the persons interviewed in that research project reported an agent called the resident and urged him to sell quickly since "people don't generally get their price once a neighborhood turns more than 50% Negro." The fear of declining property values was enough to seduce white residents into selling quickly, creating a self-fulfilling prophecy.

Because of the exclusionary practices of brokers and agents, areas where black families could live became overcrowded. In Philadelphia, for example, by 1970, areas that had transitioned from all-white to mixed housing had become virtually all-black. Zoning laws allowed single family houses to be divided up into rooming houses and spawned the proliferation of bars and clubs in those areas, which also received fewer municipal services. As a result, property values steadily decreased.[40]

Home ownership is a key contributor to family wealth. Today, white families have forty-one times more wealth than black families because, in part, roughly 72 percent of white families own their home, while 44 percent of black families own their homes.[41] Specifically, according to a recent study conducted by the Institute for Policy Studies, "the median black family today owns $3,600— just 2 percent of the $147,000 of white families."[42] Notably, wealth for the median black family dropped since the early 1980s while wealth for the median white household increased over that same period of time.[43]

By the mid-twentieth century, segregation in public education had been outlawed in Pennsylvania. However, it was still the law of the land in many other states, so collective resistance resulted in major judicial and legislative actions to decodify the centuries of discrimination and other heinous acts of racism on the books in the area of education. For example, the 1954 *Brown v. Board of Education* case[44] was filed on behalf of African American children from Kansas, South Carolina, Virginia, and Delaware who sought admission to the public schools in their community on a nonsegregated basis. Their local courts told the children they could not attend the schools, based on the *Plessy v. Ferguson*[45] decision that upheld segregation that was purportedly separate but equal. The plaintiffs' chief attorney, Thurgood Marshall, and the team of attorneys representing the plaintiffs in the Brown case challenged the *Plessy v. Ferguson* "separate but equal" doctrine head-on.

On May 17, 1954, the Supreme Court issued its first decision in the *Brown* case and held that separate educational facilities are inherently unequal, and therefore segregation in public education deprives students of equal protection of the law in violation of the U.S. Constitution. The Supreme Court reasoned that evidence from sociologists, anthropologists, psychologists, and psychiatrists established that state-imposed segregation is harmful to black children because it generates feelings of inferiority that negatively affect a student's motivation to learn.

A year later, in *Brown v. Board of Education II*[46] the Supreme Court ordered desegregation of segregated school districts and remanded the cases to the local courts that originally heard the cases to implement the decision. Charles Ogletree examined the impact of the *Brown* litigation and noted that by the mid-1970s, Supreme Court cases decided after *Brown* made it difficult to put desegregation plans into action and actually excused some predominantly white suburban school districts from their obligation to participate in desegregation plans involving urban school districts that were largely black.[47] And while some school districts were still under court desegregation orders into the twenty-first century, there has been little effort to enforce them.[48] Recent studies confirm that while there were modest gains in terms of school desegregation from the 1960s to the late 1980s, Supreme Court jurisprudence has made it easier for schools to skirt their obligations regarding desegregation, and many such programs have since been discarded. A 2012 report found that the overwhelming majority (74 percent) of black students attend schools where the majority of their peers are not white. Of black students, 38 percent attend schools referred to as "intensely segregated," in that 10 percent or less of the students enrolled are not white, and 15 percent of black students attend schools that are virtually all black. On the other hand, the typical white student attends a school where three-quarters of the students are also white.[49]

Certainly the *Brown* decisions were significant legal victories that paved the way for educational and employment opportunities for countless black people. Yet despite their purpose to remedy past discrimination, they may have been limited in terms of the benefits realized by the masses of black people. The presence of a few black students in a majority white school is a piecemeal step toward racial equality if on the whole, America's black students are going to schools that get less funding than schools attended by most of America's white students.

It was not until the 1960s that laws were passed that explicitly disapproved of discrimination in the areas of housing, recreation, employment, education, and voting rights. In 1961, for example, President John F. Kennedy signed Executive Order 10925 requiring those doing business with the government to "take affirmative action to ensure that applicants are employed, and that employees are treated during employment, without regard to their race, creed, color or national origin."[50] A decade after the *Brown* decision, the United States Congress passed the Civil Rights Acts of 1964. The events surrounding the passage of the act included an arduous battle between John F. Kennedy and Richard Nixon for president of the United States. Richard Nixon had served as President Dwight Eisenhower's vice president, and part of Kennedy's campaign strategy in 1960 was to criticize Eisenhower's position on civil rights. After Kennedy amassed support from 68 percent of African-American voters, there were tremendous expectations of the new president. However, as Barbara and Charles Whalen record in their discourse on the legislative history of the Civil Rights Act,[51] Kennedy had what he viewed as a dilemma. He stepped into a congressional arena that was predominantly conservative on behalf of a political party that, to that point, had not courted the black vote, and he was pushing a civil rights law in an environment that might cost him support and even reelection.[52] Nonetheless, in the spring of 1963, civil rights advocates, including Martin Luther King Jr., began to force Kennedy's hand. They staged large and highly publicized protests in Birmingham, Alabama, that resulted in King's imprisonment and televised police action that included police dog attacks, clubbings, and hosing of protesters, many of whom were women and children. The world was outraged, and Kennedy appeared on television and gave the speech that was the prelude to the passage of major civil rights legislation:

> We are confronted primarily with a moral issue. It is as old as the Scriptures and it is as clear as the American Constitution. The heart of the question is whether all Americans are to be afforded equal rights and equal opportunities, whether we are going to treat our fellow Americans as we want to be treated. . . . One hundred years of delay have passed since President Lincoln freed the slaves, yet their heirs, their grandsons, are not fully free. They are not yet freed from the bonds of injustice. They are not yet freed from social and economic oppression. And this Nation, for all its hopes and all its boasts, will not be fully free until all its citizens are free. Now the time has come for this Nation to fulfill its promise. It is a time to act in Congress, in your state and local legislative body and, above all, in all of our daily lives. Next week, I shall ask the Congress of the United States to act, to make a commitment it has not fully made in this century to the proposition that race has no place in American life or law.[53]

Within a little more than a week, President Kennedy presented the bill to Congress that formed the basis for what would become the Civil Rights Act of 1964, which prohibited discrimination in employment, education, and public accommodations on the basis of race and other protected characteristics such as color, religion, sex, and national origin.[54] Kennedy's suggestion that the country could somehow legislate away centuries of racial hatred and terrorism, may have been improbable, however. Even after the passage of Title VII of the Civil Rights Act of 1964, which specifically prohibited discrimination in employment on the basis of race, there remains a glaring underrepresentation of black people across a variety of professions and industries. Black workers certainly occupy many professions in greater numbers than before the passage of Title VII. Examples can be seen from the highest levels of government to the boardrooms of the country's most profitable corporations. Notably, Thurgood Marshall became the first black Supreme Court justice in 1967, and Barack Obama was the first black president of the United States in 2009. However, a review of 2017 employment statistics suggest that the law that was lauded as "a historic achievement for American society"[55] may well have been limited in terms of its application to black people. For example, while black workers make up 12 percent of the civilian labor force, less than 4 percent of persons employed in the United States as chief executives are black. Only 2.1 percent of architects, 3.7 percent of dentists, and 5.6 percent of lawyers are black.[56] Yet when you examine those positions that African Americans occupy in numbers that are disproportionate to their representation in the labor force, they remain clustered in lower paying professions with more difficult working conditions. Almost 25 percent of personal care aides, 25.5 percent of couriers and messengers, 32.3 percent of security guards and gaming survellance officers, and 28.4 percent of taxi drivers and chauffeurs are black.[57]

In 2017, the unemployment rate for black people was 7.5 percent, almost twice the unemployment rate for white people (3.8 percent). Black workers continue to earn considerably less than white workers: the median usual weekly earnings for full-time black workers was $712 compared to $937 for white workers.[58] In

2016, white families were paid about 1.7 times what was paid to black families. The white median household income was $62,769, and the black family median income was well below that at $36,615.[59]

There is probably no greater indicator of the Supreme Court's twentieth- and twenty-first-century stance on race than its activity in the area of affirmative action and education. By the early 1970s, in an effort to fulfill the aspirations and promises of equal opportunity articulated by the executive and judicial branches of government in the 1960s, many colleges had begun using race as a factor in their admissions decisions in an effort to better integrate their student bodies. However, in 1978, the Supreme Court began to set limits on what could be done to ensure equality in postsecondary education. In California, lawmakers passed a resolution that permitted the University of California to establish racial quotas. A number of lawsuits were brought against the university, but the one that the Supreme Court used to invalidate the use of racial quotas in higher education was the 1978 *Regents of the University of California v. Bakke* decision.[60] In 1973 and 1974, Allan Bakke, a white applicant for admission to the University of California at Davis Medical School, was twice denied admission. He challenged the medical school's admission program, which reserved places in each entering class for economically or educationally disadvantaged applicants and members of minority groups (which the medical school defined as African Americans, Latinos, American Indians, and Asian Americans). The court agreed with Bakke and decided that colleges could not use racial quotas in making admissions decisions.

Twenty-five years after *Bakke*, the Supreme Court looked at the issue again and decided that schools could lawfully use a program that considers race as one factor among many in an individualized consideration of each applicant.[61] In reaching its decision, the court recognized the educational benefits of a diverse student body, including preparing all students for an increasingly diverse workforce and society, cultivating leaders, breaking down stereo-types, and fostering cross-racial understanding—an understand-ing of diversity that emphasizes its benefits for white students over its advantages for a fairer society. However, the court decided that race or ethnic background could not be a decisive factor.[62]

In 2013 and again in 2016, the Supreme Court revisited the question of how a university can permissibly use race as a consid-eration in college admissions decisions.[63] The Supreme Court con-tinues to reject the use of fixed percentage admission goals for particular races and ethnicities and will only approve the use of race as a factor in admissions decisions if a university can prove that a "nonracial approach" would not produce the educational benefits of diversity "about as well and at tolerable administrative expense."[64] The use of higher education as a social tool toward racial progress has thus been formally constrained since college administrators floated the idea in the early 1970s. Notably, points for legacy, quality of high school, strength of high school curricu-lum, and standardized test scores, which very often relate to racial privilege, have not been limited or invalidated.

We have now catalogued a significant gap between the rights and privileges inherited by white and black Americans, one that has continued to grow as persistently as that growth has been resisted. And we haven't even scratched the surface of the full nar-rative and the elements of mass incarceration, voter suppression, and individualized bigotry. We have focused on just three of the interlocking structural issues—housing, education, and jobs—that get to the heart of a major cause of poverty and other quality of life issues for all people. Studies continue to confirm that higher levels of education result in a greater likelihood that an individual will be employed.[65] Individuals with higher levels of education generally get higher paying jobs than individuals with less education.[66] Businesses cluster in areas with an educated workforce to employ. But remember, K–12 education is funded based on a nineteenth-century formula of federal, state, and local resources, with the heaviest reliance on local resources collected through property taxes. Black families were legally denied equal opportunities for housing and employment until the mid-1960s and therefore were clustered for the most part in urban areas with higher rates of poverty and lower property values. They have since lagged behind their white counterparts in terms of earnings and net worth. Therefore, continuing to base a school funding system on factors like personal income, real estate value, and the corresponding ability to raise tax revenue disadvantages black students and is essentially a proxy for racism.

The 1960s did bring new approaches to education funding in the form of subsidies and add-ons available to schools for poverty, special education, and English language learners. Although a façade of benevolence is certainly created through the provision of subsidies and supplements for poverty, these supplements have been insufficient to meet the actual need of less resourced districts to educate a child living in poverty. Even with the subsidies factored in, wealthier communities in Pennsylvania, like Lower Merion, with property tax revenue supplemented by the state, were able to spend upward of $28,000 per student in 2015–2016 and are populated predominately by white students. During that same school year, Philadelphia, a school district that serves predominantly black students, spent less than half of that number, $13,880 per student.[67]

The inequity in the education system is frustratingly self-perpetuating. Education is one of the primary tools for upward mobility. The system has excluded black people from opportunities to attain the same level of education as their white counterparts to compete, and then makes the rules such that those with the most education win. As the level of achievement that a student is able to attain in a well-resourced school rises—with smaller classes, counselors, Advanced Placement courses, technology, music and arts programs, and safe facilities—this new level of achievement becomes the standard for admission to selective schools. In addition, while a number of colleges and universities no longer rely on standardized test scores in making admissions decisions, for the majority of colleges and universities, the primary basis on which admissions decisions are made is a standardized admissions test like the SAT and ACT. Expensive courses teach high school students who can afford the course how to maximize their performance on these examinations. Some well-resourced secondary schools offer a curriculum that better prepares students to perform on standardized tests. Again, the legal mandate to deny black families opportunities in housing, employment, and education resulted in these families more often than their white counterparts living in communities with fewer resources and inferior schools, housing, and jobs. The educational inequity is compounded by emerging school choice policies that let families opt out of poorly performing schools to go to better ones, leaving behind those who lack the resources to switch schools and thereby ensuring that the least resourced schools are comprised entirely of the least resourced families. Thus, even if the laws like the Civil Rights Act of 1964 require that admissions decisions be race neutral (i.e., prohibits admissions personnel from denying admission because of a student's race) yet keep in place admissions standards such as standardized test scores, the number of AP courses, and the quality of one's high school, the law has done very little to advance those who have been relegated to underresourced schools and learning environments or ensure that their children will have a better chance at accessing the resources that help American children find opportunities to secure their futures.

A 2013 study confirms that "the American postsecondary system is a dual system of racially separate and unequal institutions" with "white students increasingly concentrated, relative to population share, in the nation's 468 most well-funded, selective four-year colleges and universities while African-American and Hispanic students are more and more concentrated in the 3,250 least well-funded, open-access, two-and four-year colleges."[68] The 468 well-funded institutions spend two to five times more per student, which results in higher graduation rates, greater acceptance rates to graduate and professional school, and higher ultimate earnings, allowing their children to access schools with opportunities and resources and thereby "reinforcing the reproduction of white racial privilege."[69]

The cycle effortlessly perpetuates itself. Better educated parents can get higher paying jobs and can afford to live in communities with greater housing value and corresponding revenue from property taxes, which contribute to higher quality schools for their children, who in turn are better educated and more resourced parents for their children. Better education, better jobs, more money, more opportunities to live in better neighborhoods with better education, better jobs, more money. Conversely, inferior education leads to lower paying jobs and fewer opportunities to live in well-resourced neighborhoods with better schools.

This is the narrative that black children must know. We should not try to defend the indefensible; rather, we must help them understand that when they see black people in profound disadvantage, it is not because black people are somehow deficient. It is because we live in a society that has yet to develop into the fullness of its humanity. We must learn and teach that this racism is so deeply embedded in U.S. culture that they will surely confront its effects. And we must prepare them to navigate that experience. We must prepare every black child to deal with poverty. This is not to say that the majority of black people in the United States live in poverty; in fact, they do not. But disproportionately they do. And even those black people who don't live in poverty often are drawn to the fight on behalf of the poor. We must prepare the black child to live in a perpetual guarded state, to live with the threat that any encounter can, without provocation, turn to conflict because they are perceived as a threat, a problem, or a lesser human. Likewise, they must live with the certainty that they will be confronted with a barrage of negative and demeaning images of people who look like them in the news, on television, and at the movies. They will be consumed with the frustration and exhaustion that comes from fighting for balanced positive images that reflect the greatness of their heritage and potential. Black children must get used to seeing white people with less talent occupying positions and having opportunities to acquire wealth that far more capable black people, inheriting hundreds of years of disadvantage, have been denied. They must live with the reality that they could be further along if it weren't for the racist systems and individual acts of bigotry that have kept them behind. This chapter begins a catalogue of that history, but the list goes on and on. We must help them endure all of this without allowing resentment and anger to rob them of their own humanity. We must do right by them.

3

Too Great for Hope

What you're thinking is what you're becoming.
—MUHAMMAD ALI

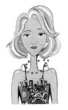 When Gabriel was four, Mike and I attempted to introduce him to a nearby soccer program. We did so with all the enthusiasm one might expect from the parents of an only-child who had only recently expressed an interest in kicking a ball into a net. After registering him and finding cleats and shin guards to match his tiny frame, we proudly brought him to a field where no less than one hundred children of all ages had also arrived to begin their season of soccer.

It was only about ten minutes into this scene that our four-year-old son observed something that we noticed but did not yet acknowledge. Twenty minutes in, he still adamantly refused to join the other kids and play. We waited him out and tried to at least get him to cheer for the other kids and learn their names. The coach, who was another kid's father, was gently persistent as he tried to coax Gabe onto the field to participate. To no avail.

After the hour was over and we drove home, my son said he didn't want to go back. A day later, we were working on some Legos together when I asked him if he still liked soccer. Without pause, he said, "Yup."

I asked, "Then why didn't you want to play on the team?"

With absolute clarity, he responded, "Because none of the other kids looked like me." And he was right.

And once again, the child shall lead them. After we confirmed that Gabe was still interested in soccer, we began to seek out opportunities that would be a better fit for our family. Another great blessing of our neighborhood and community was that we didn't need to look far before we found the Multicultural United Soccer Club, where kids as young as four and well into their teens were active, and their families had critical roles to play, from marking out the playing fields and removing rocks to coaching teams and translating any of the various languages spoken. As we had hoped, Mike and I were among only a handful of white participants and enjoyed the observable connection Gabe felt to his new team.

Karen T. Craddock will tell you the behavior I observed is part of a predictable process in our brains. Craddock's research as an applied psychologist, action researcher, and strengths-based practitioner found that, "our neurobiological network is wired to connect. Which is why belonging and exclusion fundamentally impact us as human beings. With generational experiences of social exclusion and inequity, marginalized groups experience chronic pain from being left out or treated less than that is literally registered in the brain."[1] Although I would hesitate to apply the word *exclusion* to Gabe's first experience of organized soccer, there is something of that when you do not feel you belong. The boys on the soccer field don't even have to set out to exclude Gabe. Exclusion doesn't need to be practiced in order to be felt. All they have to do is connect with the people they feel most kinship with, and at first blush, that's unlikely to be Gabe, so Gabe's going to feel left out, especially if he's experienced that before. Further, inclusion is not the absence of exclusion—it's its own practice.

Craddock goes on to explain how necessary it is to "disrupt these cycles of bias that seed empathic dysfunction" as early as we can with children. Seeing this research long after Gabe's soccer debut was helpful to give me language for what I was acting on instinctively. This was among the first of many occasions when I recognized, deeply and even painfully, what it must feel like to look different. Mike and I have had a lifetime of experiences in predominately white spaces and have never known that feeling. As a parent, it is a lot to take in, particularly when the science of it is further explained.

> A groundbreaking area of relational neurophysiology or brain science identified how social exclusion appears in the brain. Social Pain Overlap Theory (SPOT) confirmed that the pain from social exclusion and pain from physical injury or illness share the same brain pathways that register distress (Dorsal Anterior Cingulate Cortex). Whether we have been punched in the stomach or wounded by direct or indirect marginalization, our brain pathways set off an alarm that activates pain.
>
> Bottom line—images, messages, and actions, whether they are direct or indirect, that signal or shout that one is left out, not worthy or deemed "lesser than" cause real hurt to our being. These experiences of marginalization and exclusion register pain in the brain, and we experience it everywhere in our body.[2]

A significant body of research points specifically to the harm that actual or perceived discrimination does to a black child's physical health, mental health, and overall well-being. Experiences of discrimination have been linked to a range of health problems in children, including elevated systolic blood pressure, early onset of insulin resistance depression, attention-deficit/hyperactivity disorder, oppositional defiant disorder, anxiety, and low self-esteem.[3]

Even before Gabe acknowledged his discomfort with the soccer team, my first instinct as we walked hand in hand onto the field that day was to hoist him onto my hip and return to the car with an abrupt rationale that "Mama got the directions wrong, and this is not our team." I would never hesitate to exert my force when needed, particularly if I felt that it would prevent a hurt, a side-eye, or any feeling of disconnection. Even if Gabe did not feel a part of that team, he was made aware that the coach, other kids and parents wanted him to participate and have fun. Folks here were genuinely expressing to Gabe that he belonged, but it wasn't enough. The lesson for me isn't just that people should be inclusive or that this soccer club wasn't nice enough; it's that they were, and Gabe was still not comfortable. A first step for Mike and me was understanding that our child was going to identify as black and not automatically a part of the environments we may see as welcoming. A black child doesn't even need to experience explicit unwelcome for this to happen. And given the science on the experience of exclusion, we knew we needed to find communities where the psychological desire to connect with like provides him an easier path to belonging. That necessitated finding spaces with black people.

By the time Gabe was four, he had a social calendar that rivaled my college years. Enrollment in preschool and soccer created plenty of activities, and the birthday party invitations began to pour in. Every few weeks, an invitation would arrive for Gabe to jump on inflatable fun houses, swim at the Y, putt a golf ball, and build his own bear. Whatever the occasion, we said yes. Even when the parties were mostly kids from school, he would take time to warm up and ease into the festivities. At other times, he was clingy. The bear-building party for one of his white classmates bordered on painful shyness. Gabe would not leave Mike's side. He reluctantly moved along with the other kids to stuff and stitch his bear. By the time the pizza arrived, Gabe was playing with two friends, and we chalked it up to a delayed nap.

A month later, we received another party invitation to one of those climbing, jumping, and swinging places. The day of the party arrived, and I noted to Mike that this was going to be iffy because of the missed naptime again. When we arrived at the party, I scanned the room for Gabe's classmates, praying that he would ease in faster with a buddy. However, the party was already hopping with the birthday girl's family and only a couple of the girls in Gabe's class. While I was busy fretting over the fact that there were only two kids he knew there, I missed him flinging off his shoes and sprinting into the mix. Mike and I made eye contact and then proceeded to chat up the parents and other adults while keeping Gabe in our sight. He was having a ball! By the time the cake came out, we were all herded into one room. Gabe was soaked in sweat and was trying to sneak icing with some of the kids I did not know. The birthday girl was engulfed by parents, grandparents, aunts and uncles, cousins, neighbors, and a handful of school friends. Around this circle were forty people, almost all black, singing in a variety of voices; only five of us were white. Gabe enjoyed the day from start to finish; there was no clinging, no hesitation, and not a minute of coaxing needed from us. The connection was immediate, and the joy and warmth of the family's celebration embraced us. Mike and I marveled at how feelings of inclusion and exclusion for Gabe began to take shape at such a young age. This observation led Val and me to explore other settings and factors that might make a black child feel included and excluded.

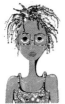 I believe Katie and Mike are among the best parents any child could have, and Katie and I agree on many things. However, an area of contention for Katie and me has been Gabe's hair. Black hair is strong. It will fight you. If not properly cared for, it will mat up, tangle up, and even break off and leave you. You can't wash it every day, and many black boys get their hair cut or groomed professionally at least every two weeks, beginning shortly after the baby boy's

first birthday, in a black barbershop. It's like a rite of passage. Growing up in Philly, I tagged along to the barbershop with my father and brother and marveled at what was behind that door flanked by the red, white, and blue barber's poles. There were good smells and creative craftsmanship, but more than that, it was a place to tell stories across generations. As they did back then, black men still take pride in being well groomed and well dressed, and they affirm each other's efforts and dreams. The more contemporary dos made popular by professional athletes are most often professionally styled. For black men, the barbershop experience feeds strong and positive cultural identity. Perhaps looking good is an in-your-face rejection of the negative images and stereotypes that portray them as shiftless, unkempt, and dreamless. I know that Gabe will be excluded from certain white communities; I simply didn't want him to also feel like an outsider in black communities. Katie and I knew all too well the reality of black children being teased for being ashy because their white parents didn't know their skin needed to be hydrated with cream daily. Gabe's hair knocked out Katie in the seventh round, and Gabe now has a nice haircut.

Both Gabe's feelings about being the only boy of color on a soccer team and his perception of his hair inform his racial identity. For decades, psychologists, sociologists, and other theorists have sought to explain racial identity using frameworks that involve movement through stages of development.[4] While these stage-based models can be helpful in understanding the ways in which some scholars believe individuals engage in a process of developing a black identity, we use the term *identity* in a broad sense to describe how black children see themselves. Scholar and Pulitzer Prize–winning author Manning Marable fleshes out the concept in a way that makes it somewhat easier to grasp.

> "Blackness" or African-American identity, however, is much more than "race." It is also traditions, rituals, values and belief systems of African-American people. It is our culture,

history, music, art and literature. Blackness is our sense of ethnic consciousness and pride in our heritage of resistance against racism.[5]

Thus, the pride that a parent can cultivate in a black child is not just a matter of race; the parent has a myriad of cultural achievements and perspectives to point to for the child to feel inspired by. Simply put, the health and well-being of black children depend on the extent to which they feel positively about being black. A poor sense of one's self as a black person results in low self-esteem and hinders the academic and personal achievement of black children.[6] Conversely, positive racial identity results in high self-esteem and academic performance, as well as a greater ability to navigate racism.[7] If parents don't work on constructing a positive black self-identity for their children, our culture will construct a negative self-identity around their blackness for them. There are at least three forces at work that threaten positive identity in black children to which we'd like to direct your attention.

The first is the creation and proliferation of negative images of black people. Underlying the stigmatization, surveillance, control, and domination of a particular group is an insidious tool of oppression—the intentional and negative distortion of the image of the group's members. If you portray a group's members in as many outlets as possible as savage, dangerous and subhuman, it will be easier to justify savagery, violence, and inhumane treatment against them, whether it's the pillage of diamonds and gold on the continent of Africa by Europeans, or slavery and discrimination in the United States. And it will be more difficult to connect and empathize with the group's members or see their contributions and value.

Here's how it works in African and African American history. In his book *The History of Africa: The Quest for Eternal Harmony*, Molefi K. Asante reminds us that many Americans perceive Africa as "helpless, stagnant or crippled in its potential" as viewed through

U.S. history books, news media, and movies.[8] In fact, Asante notes that "in the West, the ignorance of Africa is palpable, like a monster that invades our brains with disbelief, deception, and disinterest, yet is everywhere around us. We are victims of probably the most uninformed educated people in the world on the subject of Africa."[9] Through the age of exploration and continuing through modernity, European colonizers constructed a racist and unfounded idea of the indigenous peoples they encountered as existing in a state of nature that would benefit from the control that colonizers would enforce in order to take advantage of the colonized land's resources. These constructions would persist in the cultural works of the time, which continue to influence the cultural works of peoples and races throughout the world today. For example, Georg Wilhelm Friedrich Hegel, the German philosopher of the eighteenth and nineteenth centuries, claimed that Africa plays no historical part in the history of the world. Rather, he described Africa as an "undeveloped spirit" and its people as "wild," "untamed," and "barbaric," promoting a general image of Africans as magicians, sorcerers, and cannibals.[10] Further, Hegel cited only tyrannical examples of African kings and rulers and then characterized these examples as evidence of the "African spirit." Yet examples of corrupt Roman leadership were never referred to as the "Roman spirit but were seen as isolated aberrations."[11] Hegel concluded that "want of self-control distinguishes the character of the Negroes."[12] Consequently, he justified slavery and colonialism by relying on the false notion that both were necessary to humanize and save the African. He fortified this invention and dismissed any suggestion that Africans contributed to history by artificially dividing Africa into three parts: (1) Africa proper, south of the Sahara; (2) European Africa, north of the Sahara; and (3) the river region of the Nile, or Egypt.[13] This allows Europe to claim the historic achievements of Northern Africa without acknowledging the attendant influence of North Africa on the achievements of Mediterranean cultures retroactively constructed as white. Hegel specifically considered ancient Egypt as "not belonging to the African spirit" although prior to the Arab invasion of Egypt in A.D. 639, there were no Arabs in Egypt; the population was overwhelmingly black. The notion of a mixed Egypt as opposed to a black Egypt has subsequently been used to misrepresent the reality that black people were at the forefront of creating what we now popularly think of as the first great civilization. A great resource for deeper study is Ibram X. Kendi's *Stamped from the Beginning*, a chronicle of the detrimental and corrosive influences of Hegel and other architects of false African images and history.[14]

The development of positive black identity continues to be undermined by negative cultural constructions of black life. The game is the same although the players have changed. As we learned in Chapter 2, racism resulted in a U.S. system of slavery and legally mandated discrimination and oppression that produces cumulative advantage for white people and disadvantage for black people in a variety of areas including education, employment, criminal justice, and health care, and that discrimination and oppression still impact overall quality of life for most black people, even today. Identity can be shaped by the myth that behavior—namely, laziness, lack of discipline, and depravity—and not racism produced these outcomes.

The contemporary media plays a significant role in perpetuating these images. News reports exaggerate negative portrayals of black people, overrepresenting them in stories about poverty and crime and underrepresenting them in other stories.

African Americans are disproportionately represented in news stories about poverty, and these stories tend to paint a picture that is particularly likely to reinforce stereotypes and make it hard to identify with black males. For example, low-income blacks in news stories are more likely to live in slums or urban areas, as opposed to rural areas, than real-world averages would suggest; more likely be entirely unemployed and "idle" (as opposed to working); and so forth. The idle black male on the street corner is not the "true face" of poverty in America, but he is the dominant one in media portrayal.[15]

Furthermore, "blacks are overrepresented as perpetrators of violent crime when news coverage is compared with arrest rates," and black men specifically are underrepresented in their roles as parent, law enforcer, or victim.[16] A study of television and print stories in the Pittsburgh media found that over a three-month period in 2010, 86 percent of television news stories and 36 percent of print stories in the Pittsburgh media were about black males committing a crime. Less than 3 percent of the stories showed young black males (ages fifteen to thirty) involved in activities outside of crime.[17]

As a result, people often equate blackness with the weakest or most vulnerable examples. It is true that racism has resulted in black people being disproportionately clustered in adverse conditions such as poverty and incarceration. But if you depend on the media to learn about black people, *black* may mean poor to you, although the majority of black people in the United States are not poor.[18] Black may mean historyless and cultureless, although black people are rich in both. Your assumption may be that incarceration is the most probable outcome for young black men, yet there are more black men aged eighteen to twenty-four years studying on college campuses than in prison, and if you consider this same age group, the number of collegians is more than double that of those incarcerated.[19] For some people, *black* may mean dangerous and less than human. These same distortions used to justify slavery, Jim Crow, and legally mandated discrimination in the U.S. in the seventeenth, eighteenth, nineteenth, and twentieth centuries are used to justify the killing of unarmed black people at the hands of white people today. Notably, experiments confirm that white people are more likely to shoot an unarmed black male than an unarmed white male.[20] In Chapters 6 and 7, we will talk more specifically about the influence of negative images on a black child's experiences with the educational system and law enforcement, respectively.

In every age and socioeconomic group, African Americans watch more television than their counterparts in other racial and ethnic groups.[21] This creates a greater risk for racial identity formation from intentionally distorted stories, stereotypes, and other negative images of themselves in the media and popular culture. We know the more black people ingest negative media images of themselves, the lower their self-esteem.[22]

Also, black children are more easily lured into mimicking unhealthy behavior when they are told that the behavior represents them. The science backs this up. Vittorio Gallese, a neuroscientist at the University of Parma, offers, "It seems we're wired to see other people as similar to us, rather than different. At the root, as humans we identify the person we're facing as someone like ourselves."[23] Other researchers have reached the consistent conclusion that "when a stereotype becomes activated, stereotype-consistent behavior may follow automatically from that activation."[24] When black children see negative images of themselves, there is a real and substantial risk that they will copy the behavior. The negative impact of the distortion is magnified if the black child has little or no real-life experiences with black people that provide counter images.

The absence of positive racial identity also can result in the development of self-hatred. I would dare to say that most black people hate the negative images they see of themselves in the media. However, those with a limited knowledge and underdeveloped understanding of their history and culture may believe that these negative characterizations are true, innate, and sweeping. They may internalize the hatred and reject everything black. They may consciously isolate themselves, choosing to be one of very few black persons in their home, work, and religious and recreational spaces. They may do everything in their power to separate themselves from anything related to black culture and do their best to look and act in a way that reflects white culture. But they may struggle to feel equitable acceptance in these contexts and end up in a vicious cycle of struggling to escape their internalized inferiority. Self-hatred leads to psychological distress and deprives the individual of the benefits of black networks, an effective source of support and connection for well-being.

They also may see themselves as an exception to what they believe is the general negative character of black people. This leads them to put pressure on themselves and others to constantly act as representatives of a better version of blackness: an unfair position to be in, a stigmatizing view to take against manners of self-expression, and a white supremacist standard to judge someone by. They tend to be ignorant of the realities of racism and somewhat unforgiving. Consequently, they blame and seek to destroy any black person who embarrasses them or threatens their black idea.

Self-hatred and poor racial identity can make it challenging for black people to see other black people as people, and easier to see them only as a good or bad image to be protected or destroyed. Without the proper perspective on racial identity, black children may grow up learning to respond to other black people by seeking to destroy the ones they believe represent a bad image or simply reveling in the virtues of the good, never learning how to engage in a process of analyzing the obstacles to racial equity. We are capable of being our own toughest critics, but we help neither ourselves nor others when we do. For example, supporting policies that lock up those most impacted by racism—black people who have been denied the educational and job opportunities to earn family sustaining wages and who are relegated to communities ravaged by concentrated poverty—instead of fighting for policies that guarantee those educational and economic opportunities has never been in the best interests of black people.

Katie knows that she and her family will need to work to help Gabriel develop positive black identity so that he becomes a confident self-advocate.

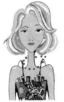 A second threat to the positive racial identity of a black child was discussed more fully in Chapter 2: the operation of systems that intentionally disadvantage black people while ensuring that white people continue to enjoy its privileges. All people need surroundings that are pleasing, strong and positive relationships, and good work (productivity) for overall well-being. Systems that relegate black people to neighborhoods that are intentionally underresourced and blighted, a biased criminal justice system whose rules disproportionately incarcerate black men thereby tearing black families and communities apart, inadequate education and limited employment opportunities for black people that impede productivity— these work together to undermine positive racial identity and well-being. "But," you say, "our family is middle class or upper middle class, and we are grateful that our child can enjoy the fruits of our privilege."

White parents of black children may themselves function as a third threat to their child's development of a positive black identity. They may dismiss the need to concern themselves with racial identity if their children enjoy a middle-class or upper-middle-class lifestyle. Frequently, white people ascribe visible inequalities in their communities to issues of class and choose not to engage with the role race has played in the allocation of a community's resources. Gabe lives in a well-appointed home in a clean and visually pleasing neighborhood, is supported by a loving family, and is in the second grade at a well-resourced school. None of these things in and of themselves are enough to give him racial pride, which we know is tied to his achievement and well-being. Therefore, we still must actively and intentionally build racial identity.

Chad Goller-Sojourner, a black adult transracial adoptee, is often asked to write and speak on this very topic. "I can't tell you how often I hear white adoptive parents say 'Well, we don't have anything around. We live in a rural community. The closest black person is three hours away.' People will fly across the country for a job. If their kid is a track star, they'll find the best school district for that before they even call the realtor. There's something about transracial adoption where people won't find a way to work it out."[25] Like it or not, this is what the National Association of Black Social Workers was attempting to guard against in 1972. Their position was that black children should be raised by black parents because white parents were ill equipped to mirror the perceptions, attitudes, and behaviors necessary for a black child's survival in a racist world, let alone that which is critical for healthy racial identity formation.

Even more, what does it say to our children when we make choices (or fail to) that do not intentionally recognize, celebrate, and mirror their racial identity? It reinforces the notion that there is one standard, universal, and superior way of being that is white or European. In fact, white parents may not even think in terms of their own racial identity or understand the need to acknowledge different racial identities. They may assume their own identity is tied to individualism or the universal human experience, not realizing that it too is shaped by race. Many white people tend to think of identity as individual. White people who think of themselves as a group are the white supremacists and nationalists, this thinking goes. This line of thinking is convenient because it lets white people off the hook from having to grapple with the messy meaning of white identity. But the reason they can get comfort from thinking of their identity as purely individual is that the world around us has normalized white culture and treated it as normal, if not universal. Many white people think of themselves as mere individuals in the world without racial identity, and they wonder why that doesn't work for everyone, but in fact they are individuals operating within a white identity that they mistake for the world. The confusion comes from the privilege of seeing white identity everywhere around them and so incorrectly assuming that it is an absence of race identity and not its own racialized group identity. A resource that we will encourage in Chapter 6, on education, is *The Guide for White Women Who Teach Black Boys*.[26] Ali Michael's chapter on white racial development is especially meaningful here. In order to fully embrace the development of positive racial identity in our black children, white parents cannot dismiss the importance of their own positive racial identity.

The promising news is that there are as many effective strategies to develop positive racial identity as there are threats to it. However, the racial mirrors held up for black children must be thoughtfully intended and selected. The consequences of hoping they see themselves positively or feel like they belong are just too great for hope.

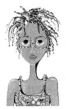 The endgame is correcting a belief in the superiority of one race over another and concurrently ridding ourselves of the pride of domination and control. This requires a recognition that white people's worldview—their culture, history, and value system—is one among many, and it is not entitled to supersede the variety of perspectives in which people might proudly center themselves. This simple but revolutionary perspective was given a theoretical framework, practical application, and a significant voice by Molefi K. Asante. With his first publication in 1980, *Afrocentricity: The Theory of Social Change*, Asante sparked an international conversation about questions of African identity, history, and culture. He coined the term *Afrocentricity* to express an idea that for African or black people, African interests, values, and perspectives should predominate. The African diaspora need not choose to center a white perspective. Afrocentricity does not espouse domination

and instead recognizes the right of Europeans to have a perspective, but as one among many, and perhaps not always the wisest. Therefore, Afrocentricity fundamentally is different from Eurocentrism, which imposes itself as universal.[27]

Katie and I both love live theater. Therefore, to further explain, we'll use the theater as metaphor. Black people are not minor characters on the periphery of a story about white or European experiences. Their stories are the central plots of different plays, unfolding on stages in theaters near and far away. All of us are central characters in different but equally powerful stories that are rich in history and culture. And while Shakespeare may be up for a Tony Award for best writer (if the Tonys had such a category), so would Cesaire, Hurston, and Soyinka. And while Bach may be recognized for his musical brilliance, so would Ellington and Coltrane. In the end, we are collectively striving to accept our racial differences "as part of a constellation of differences rather than assuming a superior place among them."[28]

Shielding black children from negative messages while saturating them with positive counterimages also have been found to be effective in building positive black identity and self-esteem while reducing the negative impact of racism on identity development.[29] For black children, that means a correct understanding of who they are and where they have come from. Become familiar with the work of Cheikh Anta Diop and other scholars that shatters the Eurocentric historical paradigm and establishes that ancient Egypt was a black civilization and Africa "stands at the very beginning of the origin of humanity."[30] Walk them through the chronology of Africa, which includes the creation of languages, the building of pyramids, and the rise of great dynasties.[31] It's the difference between telling black children they started this life as enslaved captives picking tobacco on a Virginia plantation or as kings and queens who built the first pyramids. Create and digest works that inspire productivity. In addition to the books already referenced, make *The History of*

Africa and *The African American People: A Global History* a part of your home library to help black children understand that despite every human effort to destroy their potential and deny their humanity, both on the continent of Africa and throughout the African diaspora—whether in Brazil, the United States, South America, the Caribbean, or Europe—black people around the world have made invaluable contributions to history. Remind them of truths: hundreds of thousands of black soldiers fought in the Revolutionary and Civil Wars, Benjamin Banneker invented the first clock made in America, and Charles Drew, M.D., developed pioneering enhancements to blood preservation techniques.

The consciousness with which we tell the story makes all the difference. Recognizing and exposing suffering is one aspect of consciousness; however, it shouldn't stop there, although many well-intentioned persons do. When the filmmaker, songwriter, or television producer presents images of black people living in neighborhoods ravaged by violence, poverty, and despair without a discussion of centuries of discrimination in education, housing, and employment, it creates an impression that the outcomes have been produced by behaviors like laziness, lack of discipline, and immorality. Speak, act, and create in a way that demonstrates an understanding of the racist systems that have worked to create concentrated poverty and hopelessness. But don't stop there. It is possible to simultaneously offer awareness of the overwhelming obstacles and hope for overcoming them by seeking out creative works and other information that demonstrate "victorious consciousness." A term coined by Asante, victorious consciousness, is moving beyond the observation of a bad condition and its cause. It is also operating with an awareness that a victorious outcome is nonetheless achievable. We lean on Asante's writing once again for an illustration.

> The victorious attitude shows the Africans on the slave ship winning. It teaches that we are free because we choose to be

free. Our choice is the determining factor, no one can be your master until you play the part of slave. Speak victoriously, dispense with resignation, create excellence, and establish victorious values. Know your history and you will always be wise. The Africans on the slave ships won in more ways than they lost. Affection, courage, and humor in their pain were the elements which gave us the right to be new people today.[32]

Visit African American museums and libraries that tell this story. There are museums dedicated to preserving African American history and culture in many U.S. cities.[33]

Foster an appreciation of African and African American culture represented in music, dance, art, literature, and most important in a value system. The question is often asked, Is there in fact an African culture? People of African descent do share a common experience, struggle, and origin. Out of that, a distinct value system and culture has emerged. African philosopher Kwame Gyekye believes that "there is no need to generalize a particular philosophical position for all African people in order for that position to be African."[34] Gyekye recognizes that cultural unity does not come from exactness in every aspect of every African civilization. Rather, the system emanates from African life and thought—basically, its beliefs, customs, traditions, values, sociopolitical institutions, and historical experiences.[35] Therefore, while there is great diversity among Africans, there are certain shared qualities across the continent and throughout the diaspora. And the diversity of that experience is part of its strength. Notably, African Americans have retained much of African culture. The retention of many cultural traditions may be due to the fact that Africans, since their arrival in the Americas and for centuries thereafter, have been segregated from others in the American population and therefore were left to practice and perpetuate many of these African traditions. Others are much more intentional about retaining African culture and passing on vital cultural traditions through rituals and practices like Kwanzaa, an annual end-of-year celebration of black culture, family, and community.[36] There are any number of ways to experience empowering African American culture. Just to name a few more, take an African dance class, listen to jazz, attend cultural festivals like Odunde in Philadelphia, read a book by Dorothy West, and see a performance by the Alvin Ailey American Dance Theater. The African American Literature Book Club provides an excellent list of African American children's books.[37]

Culture also includes a group's perspectives and values. In the United States, the white or European way of being is considered by many Americans as the standard, and they have little or no knowledge that another perspective or African worldview exists. This is not to suggest that the concepts put forth are exclusive to African people. Gyekye explains that "describing a body of ideas as African is not in the sense that these ideas are not to be found anywhere else in the world, but in the sense that this body of ideas is seen, interpreted, and analyzed by many African thinkers (and societies) in their own way."[38] Below are just two of the many shared African cultural values.

Good Equals Beautiful

Aesthetic is the standard by which something is judged or evaluated as beautiful. Some theories of aesthetics deal only with physical beauty. In the African tradition, however, notions of beauty are grounded in quality, and it is difficult to discuss beauty in terms of physicality: body size and type, hair texture, skin tone, and the size and shape of facial features. This concept is embodied in the African term *Nzuri,* which means what is good is beautiful and what is beautiful is good. There is no separation of the two. Nothing is beautiful in and of itself, but because it does good. It is grounded in some aspect of the community; it is participatory. Similarly, to be a good person, you must do good things. In Akan communities, the sole criterion for goodness is the welfare of the community. Consequently, good deeds such as kindness and truth-fulness promote human well-being. On the issue of justice, there are no winners and losers. The key principle is not to humiliate others, and everyone is to be treated with dignity and respect. Similarly, with respect to oppression, the African concept runs counter to that of the West. According to African tradition, if the oppressed are liberated, everyone is liberated because the oppressor no longer lives to control the oppressed but can live freely, thereby increasing and becoming more honorable. In such a system, oppressors cannot be said to be free just as the oppressed cannot. You can demonstrate alignment with these values by supporting national efforts to dismantle oppressive systems like the Equal Justice Initiative or local efforts like the Public Interest Law Center in Philadelphia.

For those of us who live in America, our children must still operate in a space where others view beauty only in the physical sense. For white parents, particular standards of beauty, like body size and type, may be associated with social status and acceptance, while others are associated with negative traits such as lack of success or discipline. Black people don't generally accept white American beauty standards such as women being thin and angular. Rather, for women, black culture tends to consider figures with curves desirable. Supporting and nurturing a child's positive racial identity may mean discarding one group's notion of beauty and celebrating the beauty that is uniquely theirs.

Similarly, there are numerous hairstyles that are compatible with a black girl's hair texture. Hairstyles typically worn by white girls are not the universal standard and may not be appropriate for a black girl's hair. Find styles that complement your child's hair texture. Look and ask for help if you need it. There are a number of excellent hair care resources for white parents, including a hair school.[39] Above all, a black child must never be left to feel that they are a failed effort to look like their white parents simply because their parents have only ever known one standard for beauty.

Communality

Communalism or communality is another African value. It empha-sizes the activities of the group over the individual. The system does not negate individual achievement but recognizes that the greatest individual achievement is that which contributes to the progress of the entire group. Otherwise, the system cannot be con-sidered a good or sophisticated system. African proverbs reflect similar sentiments:

> *"One finger cannot lift up a thing."*
> *"If one man scrapes the bark of a tree for medicine, the pieces*
>   *fall down."*
> *"The left arm washes the right arm, and the right arm washes*
>   *the left."*

As we discussed in the introduction, in traditional African cul-tures, there was no concept of the nuclear family; the community formed the basis for the family unit, and biology was often less important than relationship. Generally, African parents do not view themselves as owners of their children; rather, parents are custodians of the gift of children. Communality is also apparent in the African and African American call-and-response ritual. Call-and-response takes place when the lead speaker makes a point and the audience responds to the point, most often with phrases demonstrating affirmation. This, in turn, empowers the speaker to connect even further with the audience. The call-and-response, which confirms the relationship between the individual and the community, figures most prominently in the black church.

While spiritual development is vital for Katie and me, and we believe that the most important role of an adult in the lives of chil-dren is to give them the tools and encouragement to develop spiri-tually, our suggestion that families with black children visit black churches is also about exposure to black culture. Black churches are rich in African cultural retentions and traditions. Chief among them is call-and-response. It is a phenomenon involving the speaker and the congregation that is so routine as to be considered custom. It allows an audience to respond to the speaker in the moment. In the context of the African American church experience, the affirmation most often takes the form of clapping or shouts to the preacher—"Amen," "Yeah," or "That's right." Yes, in the moment. In *The Music of Martin Luther King, Jr.,* Richard Lischer draws the parallel between African and African ritual in terms of call-and-response:

> The key to any black preacher's style is the responsiveness of the congregation. The call-and-response pattern dates back to the West African ring shout and to the earliest forms of worship among African Americans. Call and response is a metaphor for the organic relations of the individual to the group in the black church.[40]

The energy from the congregation fuels the preacher so that their oratory becomes increasingly ardent. Underlying this ritual is the notion that the preacher and people share the space, the information, and the experience. Many European-styled presentations tend to be more individualistic. The speaker is considered to own the space and content, which they impart to a waiting audience. The audience doesn't see themselves as co-owners of the presentation or content and therefore refrains from interrupting the presentation and reserves any engagement until the conclusion of the presentation, expressing their gratitude generally by clapping.

In addition to whether Gabe should get regular haircuts, Katie and I disagreed on how to respond to public speakers outside of the church. When workshop speakers and other presenters begin their speeches with the customary salutation "Good morning," I am often one of only a few black people in the room who respond out loud in kind with "Good morning!" Katie invariably looks at me and rolls her eyes. As the speaker moves into the formal presentation, if something particularly poignant is said, I affirm and encourage the speaker with either a head nod or perhaps a short verbal affirmation. That will surely prompt another eye-roll from Katie and her reminder to me in a stern whisper that "everything is not a black Baptist church experience." My explanations of the differences between European and African culture fell on deaf ears. We went on like this for years. But one day, it all changed.

Mike, Katie, Gabe, and I visited the Catholic church where one of our priest friends serves as pastor. Katie was very comfortable in the space because she grew up Catholic; however, this was a black Catholic church with a black priest. What she didn't know was that many black Catholic churches with black priests resemble black Baptist churches in worship style if not in length of service. And then it happened. Whenever a speaker said, "Good morning!" everyone responded back, "Good morning!" Then the drum and piano rhythms permeated the grand and lofty structure. People were standing and clapping and responding orally and loudly. I looked at Katie, and she was trying her best to hold back. But I could see it was getting good to her. At first she moved her head back and forth. I think I may have heard an audible noise; it sounded more like a grunt than a word. But she would not relent and give up anything audible. I looked over again, and her left hand was slapping her left thigh as her head bopped. She was all in during the nearly two-hour service.

Our next church experience together was at the wedding of a coworker. At a black church. From the first note, it was clear that the soloist was going to wreck the place. Her voice was soul-stirring. The mostly black audience was engaged and affirming. I looked over at Katie, and she too was engaged and affirming. She had done what Goller-Sojourner wishes more white adoptive parents would do: "If you admit that it would be uncomfortable for you to move, to go to a black church, or do your grocery shopping on the other side of town, then I say, if somebody is going to be uncomfortable better you than the children."[41] Katie had intentionally submitted herself to a process of discomfort for Gabe and emerged on the other side if not with a greater level of comfort, then certainly with a greater level of understanding.

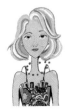With positive racial identity, a black child need not be hindered by the physical pain and psychological distress of exclusion and low self-esteem, nor be gripped with anxiety, plagued by poor health outcomes, or discouraged under the weight of self-hatred. Rather, children can be motivated in a positive direction by the reality of vast possibilities. It is critical for Mike and me that Gabe is taught about race in a way that is most empowering for him, that he sees things in a way that provokes him to work for racial equity, and that he measures his success not just by the rungs of the ladders he is able to climb but by the number of people he helps to join him on the ladder. But this is not simply a matter of hoping for a good outcome. It is a matter of intentionally doing those things that foster positive racial identity in children. What I know is that I owe Gabe that and more. We will inspect and explore together while keeping one another close. We will question and test and give others a chance to support us and join us. We will do this together.

4

In Living Color

Your child should not be your first black friend.
—CHAD GOLLER-SOJOURNER

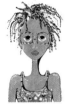Living communally has always made sense to me. Perhaps it is because my mother died when I was young, and I had to depend on older cousins, aunts, grandmothers, the mothers of my friends, teachers, and other women in my community to model behavior for me. I had great parents, but there were others around me who did not. Even as a child, what made the most sense to me was for adults around children to stand in the gap for parents who were unavailable or unable to parent well. And even if parents were well resourced and well equipped, they never seemed able to do everything and appeared to benefit from the support of an extended community. Many who have closely examined the issue agree with the instincts of my youth: children benefit when they are loved and supported by different relationships—grandparents, aunts and uncles, coaches, neighbors, and family friends.[1]

When I talk to white parents of black children, many express a desire to cultivate a community that includes adults who look like their black child and can share the load of helping to nurture healthy and positive racial identity in their child. However, most white families live in predominantly white neighborhoods, send their children to predominantly white schools, and carry out their religious beliefs in predominantly white places of worship.[2] So the question I get most often is, "How do I build this diverse community?" Katie and I refuse to belittle the question because we believe the desire is real and the task for some is intimidating. "How do I make black friends?" they ask. Our response: Intentionally. Desiring and then working toward a particular outcome are the first steps in seeing the outcome realized. And because we believe a successful outcome will ultimately benefit children, we eagerly share our best advice and a part of our story with the hope that parents are inspired to move forward with building an intentional village.

1. **You will need context.** Very often, a space to encounter persons of different races presents itself without much effort. You work in a diverse workplace or you live in a diverse neighborhood. But more often, people function in segregated spaces. They go to an all-white or all-black place of worship, live in a neighborhood with people who look like them, and socialize with people who look like them. For white parents of black children, you must go where black people are. Volunteer at a church or other nonprofit organization that works on issues of interest to black people. Move to a neighborhood where black people also live. Be willing to endure the discomfort of being in a space where everyone doesn't look like you so your child can have the comfort of seeing other people who look like them. If you do this, there will likely be ample opportunities for interactions with a black coach, teacher, or spiritual leader, or the parents of your child's friends. While these role models are important and can provide you with helpful advice and guidance, these relationships may not automatically develop into close friendships that provide a

deeper constant in your child's life. Many white parents tell us they want that deeper connection.

2. **You have to want to know someone and be known to them.** Like any relationship, going beyond superficial interactions to friendship requires a desire to want to know someone and to also be known to others. This means taking the time and making the effort to know what a black person's world is like and what issues are important to black people as a community. It goes beyond admiration for black public figures who have courted a white audience such as politicians, professional athletes, and entertainers. It means familiarizing yourself with black intellectual and philosophical thought. Your interests and values will not line up with everyone regardless of race or ethnicity, and closer friendships may not be appropriate or forthcoming. However, if those interests and values do line up, be willing to invest the time and energy it takes to get to know a person as an individual and to be known by the person. It is not as an ego exercise to show the world how enlightened you are for having secured a black friend but rather because of a genuine desire to know other people and what makes them tick, as well as to share some of yourself with them.

3. **Sow into their interests and dreams.** We are all gifted with wonderful and extraordinary attributes. But we need others in order to develop and mature in them. Sometimes we stand still or go backward because we are not encouraged enough in our dreams. Other times we forge ahead too quickly and dogmatically, leaving casualties in our path. Or we can go sideways, veering off the course of what we set out to do. Friends show an interest in what is important to the other, they remind each other that they are wonderfully

made, they challenge and encourage each other, and they celebrate even small victories as we grow in the areas that yearn for development.

To better illustrate our point, here's a bit of our story.

Katie and I met at Temple University. Katie's first position at Temple was in the division of student affairs, the arm of the university that supports the personal development of college students. Professionals in this field provide students with guidance and services in a range of areas, including orientation to college life, leadership development, student government, disability resources, behavioral health, recreation, and discipline. I was one of the university's lawyers, and student affairs was among my areas of responsibility, so Katie would routinely consult with me for legal advice.

Of all the aspects of Katie's job, she was most drawn to the student discipline process, which she managed. At times, a college student's conduct may constitute a violation of the university's code of conduct, but it could simultaneously be charged as a crime under the state's criminal law. On these occasions, a student may need to secure an attorney to prepare for a case, and that would require that I be involved. This was our context.

Step two was getting to know Katie and learning what drives her. Katie's interest in the interpretation of the university's policies and the state law was insatiable. Katie had a particular devotion to students who might be navigating the process without proper support or advice and would do all she could to ensure that students were properly supported and afforded a fair and equitable process. While the context of our meeting was our shared workplace, Katie was drawn to the legal profession and engaged me in frequent discussions about the wisdom and justness of laws and policies. We shared all the important core values, so after we checked those boxes, we could move on and gradually learn more about each other.

Step two also involved learning what inspires Katie and who she aspires to be. It came as no surprise to me that Michelle Obama is Katie's spirit guide. Katie more than adores the former first lady, and she was giddy when her book, *Becoming*, came out in 2018. Katie called me when she first cracked open the autobiography to read her favorite parts aloud. "I spent much of my childhood listening to the sound of striving. It came in the form of bad music, or at least amateur music, coming up through the floorboards of my bedroom—the *plink plink plink* of students sitting downstairs at my great-aunt Robbie's piano, slowly and imperfectly learning their scales."[3] Katie would exclaim, "Don't you just love her!" That was not posed as a question; it was an emphatic statement. Then she would gleefully point to a similarity: "I had a great Aunt Bobbie with a giant piano in her house!" I see these two women as sharing more than beloved elderly aunts.

Most people in this country have only known or observed the former first lady as the steadfast wife of the first African American president of the United States and mother to two beautiful daughters who would be required to navigate their growth and development inside of the White House and under an often cruel and skeptical microscope. For Michelle Obama to allow herself, her life, and her history to be known, especially to a country that did not always embrace her or her story, was a demonstration of the kind of courage that Katie holds in the highest regard, particularly because Mrs. Obama supported a political life that she did not choose. As a graduate of Princeton followed by Harvard Law, Michelle had her own career, which was never intended to include politics. Before her husband's future office really took hold, Michelle Obama decided to leverage her power, influence, network, and resources to serve her home community in Chicago and later develop a platform as first lady to advocate for children, education, nutrition, and military families. In the multitude of ways that the first lady intentionally made the White House accessible to all—planting a garden, music concerts, Girl Scout sleepovers,

Mom Dancing with Jimmy Fallon on *The Tonight Show*—Katie believes that Michelle exemplified the importance of children and people of all races, creeds, and colors feeling like the nation's capital was theirs. Katie couldn't get enough of her untypical FLOTUS coverage rapping—"This is For My Girls. All around the world. Stand up. Put your hands up. Don't take nothin' from nobody"— with Missy Elliott and James Corden, yet another sign that the White House was accessible to everyone. Perhaps this commitment to authenticity was nurtured in the first lady by her father, who taught her the same core principles that Katie's father emphasized for her path: to work hard, laugh often, and keep your word, and that your story is what you have and will always have, so it must be something you own.

I know that Katie's aspirations align with Michelle Obama's fierce partnership with her husband, her unfailing strength for her daughters, and her devotion to her mother and brother. Family comes second to nothing. Both Michelle and Katie show up in that way for marriage, motherhood, their own mothers, and their siblings. Katie even shows up when she is the only white person at my ninety-six-year old aunt's funeral in the hood! Katie's brand of reliability makes our friendship a special gift.

Katie does have an eye to emulate Michelle Obama's style and elegance in fashion, and she is inspired by the way the first lady is poised and careful with her words yet never shies away from stating truth. For all those who clamored to call the 2008 election the mark of a postracial America, FLOTUS inserted truth into the narrative by reminding the world that she wakes up every day in a house built by enslaved Africans. Katie also feels compelled to point out injustices when they need attention and is relent-less when it comes to making her case. She is straight-talking, no-nonsense, and devoted to improving the lives of others. Her calling is significant and can at times be overwhelming.

While our formula is not perfectly linear, step three—sowing into another person's interests and dreams—is essential. Friendship is rarely a one-way street. The way I try to support Katie is to make what may seem too big smaller or funnier. One of Katie's responsibilities at Temple was to organize a series of activities to welcome more than five thousand new students and their parents. It was a big and stressful task. The welcome week activities culminated in a huge cookout, which also was Katie's responsibility. While Katie is energized by a project she can sink her teeth into, too many people and loose ends can be distressing. I headed over to the cookout to see if I could help. She was tired and looked as much. As we walked across campus and she was rattling off the latest three things that didn't come off as planned, a young man hollered out to Katie, "Hey sexy!" Now, Katie can put it together with the best of them and rock a tailored suit, pearls, and stilettos with ease, but on this day, she had not put it together. As I scanned her seventies-style burgundy cotton wrap skirt (it was 2006) and flip-flops (not the Tory Burch or Ferragamo type), I said, "These kids smoke too much." We howled with laughter for what seemed like an hour.

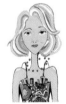 Knowing Val also involves knowing a former first lady. Val was actually born two days after Eleanor Roosevelt died, and sometimes I think she thinks she's the black reincarnation of the former first lady. Val's mother died when Val was just eleven; Eleanor Roosevelt's mother died when she was eight. Both Val and Eleanor were raised by fathers whom they adored. Val admires Eleanor Roosevelt primarily because despite her foibles, when Eleanor had an opportunity or a platform, she demonstrated the courage to take a stand on racial issues and challenge the world's prevalent views on racial equity and justice. In 1939, the Daughters of the American Revolution (a group of blue-blooded white women) refused to allow the prominent black singer Marian Anderson to perform at Washington's Constitution Hall. As a result, the first lady resigned

from her membership in the group and used her role and influence to arrange for Miss Anderson to sing instead on the steps of the Lincoln Memorial. She did this in a big and very public way to expose the smallness and bigotry of the organization while elevating the tremendous creative talent, poise, and grace of Miss Anderson to the world.

Val admires how instrumental Eleanor Roosevelt was in support of the civil rights movement, particularly her sophisticated instinct for using the media and press corps to illuminate the message she wanted to highlight. One such example that Val will frequently call upon was a now famous photograph that captured Eleanor's brilliant smile while she was seated next to Tuskegee Airman Charles Alfred Anderson, a black man, in 1941. When black men were training to be military aviators in the U.S. Armed Forces, Jim Crow laws still segregated service men and prevented black aviators from serving as fighter pilots. With her press crew in tow, the First Lady seized the opportunity to visit the Tuskegee Air Corps Flight School in Alabama, where black pilots were trained, for more than just a tour of the facility. She also went for a thirty-minute flight with Chief Flight Instructor Anderson. The press corps photo and quotable endorsement of Chief Anderson gave extensive exposure to the demon of racism and the deficit to the country it caused. Val believes that incident was a positive step toward racial integration in military service.

This story has a special place in Val's heart because her own father served in a segregated Army infantry unit in the South Pacific during World War II and, decades later, her brother attended Tuskegee University. And while we all have some platform—certainly most are not as big as Eleanor Roosevelt's—Val believes that when she has a platform, whether it is a board room, the classroom, a small social event, or a one-on-one encounter, she should be able to articulate a position that encourages progress toward racial equity. She's committed to the message and loves its various forms. She admires those who can effectively use comedy and is captivated by blazing oratory. But for Val, she wants to be able to articulate the message with such precision and warmth that it goes down easy. She wants people to get it, to see the humanity of the most marginalized, the ills of conventional systems, and the greater potential in all of us. Actually, one of the highest compliments Val received was when a local radio host, after wrapping up an interview she gave him on air, told her he couldn't wait to book her again on another topic because her voice was "like syrup."

There is no question that I admired Val before I even really got to know her. That syrup that she can pour out is always impressive, particularly because it always appears to effortlessly improve upon any subject. Whether it was her keynote for a "prestigious women in leadership" event, her acceptance speech when recognized by the Barrister's Association, or her instruction to fellow congregants who participate in Bible study with her, Val's level of reflection, preparation, and practice is the same. Val is relentless in her application of syrup. To know her enthusiasm for preparation is not only daunting but hilarious. From the moment I find out that another fabulous invitation has been extended to Val, I begin my incessant teasing about what draft she is on and reminding her to turn off Track Changes of her own edits. And while there is certainly nothing wrong with preparation and wanting to do your best, I never let her take her task too seriously. That's how I do step three and support her as my friend. On the surface, it would appear that someone so talented and accomplished wouldn't need anything, yet part of getting to really know friends and being known to them includes figuring out how they would like to be supported.

Consequently, whatever vetting Val put me through, she trusted me enough to share all that she was investing into feeling prepared. This could include a midday phone call of "Hey, gurl, whatcha doin'? I have this thing coming up, and I need you to take a look at what I have written so far," followed by hours and hours of her privately reading, polishing, and memorizing. Next, there might be spontaneous pop-ins, legal pad in hand, where Val tests some examples and ideas to see where they land with an audience, namely me. When the big event arrives—in her circles, these events are big—she has somehow scored me a ticket to attend, which gives me the chance to be her wingwoman and finesse any details that the host may have forgotten. The eternal student in Val has, in recent years, taken to the idea of me recording her delivery for deconstruction later. All of this occurs whether the audience is a room full of the one percenters or a handful of eighth graders. The precision of language, selection of stories or anecdotes to make meaning for her listeners, the rhythm and seamlessness of message, and call to action are all ingredients to her syrup recipe.

Val and I had been remarkably good friends for a few years when Mike and I shared that we had started the process to become eligible adoptive parents. Our process included providing three support letters from nonfamily, and Val was a perfect choice. Among the many questions and probings about ourselves and how we planned to raise a child was the critical section about whom we believed we could adopt. More specifically, we needed to identify the race or races of a child whom we would consider adopting. Mike and I dialogued and prayed often about each phase of becoming paper-ready prospective adoptive parents, and we sought out members of our constructed community to join us. Even before we knew about Gabriel, Val and I were in frequent and deep contemplation of all that would be necessary to parent a child of a different race. Knowing Val, this was more than her sowing her wisdom into me; it was the beginning of her sowing her wisdom into our future family.

As soon as Val knew that Gabriel was on his way home to Pennsylvania with us, Aunt VaVal (her appointed name once he could speak) was in full force. The gifts of clothes and books, the hours of cuddling and rocking, and the stern and emphatic lectures on how important all this attention and doting and loving on Gabe in the first thirty-six months of life would be for his development (of course she had consulted the latest research on the issue) were part of our new normal. When we opened one of her frequent and generous gifts (from a high-end boutique that imprints their boxes and wraps each article in delicate paper) and held up this latest outfit with matching shoes, I could not help but gasp. When he was six months old, I could barely keep socks on his feet, let alone these fancy brand kicks that were barely four inches long. As my eyes had just rolled halfway back, Val swiftly declared, "You will not have my nephew in mismatched track suits and slipper socks." Seven years later, Gabe is smart, eye-catchingly attractive, and extremely confident. When girls who are two and three years older than Gabe pay him more attention than I feel necessary, or he revels in dishing out some quick-witted response that belies his age, Val will turn to me, roll her eyes, and acknowledge, "Okay, maybe we overdid it in those first thirty-six months."

Life calls for the best of what we all bring, and we need others to help us be our best. While I am a fighter, I can rely on Val to remind me that some situations are more nuanced and complicated than I see and may require a kinder, more measured and strategic approach. I revel in reminding Val to set limits on those things and people she can help so as not to neglect and deplete herself.

While Val and I can imagine the other as Michelle Obama and Eleanor Roosevelt, in reality we're probably more like Lucy Ricardo and Ethel Mertz. But we see each other as so much more than we really are and that has been one of the great gifts of our friendship. Our sincere hope is that by exposing our aspirations, flaws, and vulnerabilities, we inspire you to engage in an introspective process as well—one that positions you to confidently forge connections with black identity and community.

5

Black Out

> One of the most frustrating features of being
> black in this country is the ongoing demand
> and effort to convince white people that what is
> happening to us is actually real.
>
> —EDDIE GLAUDE JR.[1]

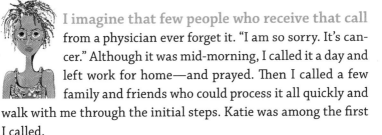 I imagine that few people who receive that call from a physician ever forget it. "I am so sorry. It's cancer." Although it was mid-morning, I called it a day and left work for home—and prayed. Then I called a few family and friends who could process it all quickly and walk with me through the initial steps. Katie was among the first I called.

Within just a few hours, my cell phone rang. "Val, I've taken a look at everything; understand that this is curable. The tumor in your lung is indolent. Stage 1A. Meet me tomorrow at 2:00, and I'll introduce you to the chief of thoracic surgery. I'll do the surgery with him." The voice on the other end of the phone was the dean of Temple University's Medical School and president and CEO of Temple's Health System, who also happened to be a thoracic surgeon. It didn't get any better than that. Friends at work reached out to him once they got word of the diagnosis.

I hung up, googled *indolent tumor*, and prayed some more. Katie would accompany me to Temple Hospital's Lung Center the next day. Located in one of Philadelphia's poorest neighborhoods, Temple Hospital is considered the city's substitute for a public hospital.

Temple Hospital's patients are predominantly black and Latinx, and 75 percent of its gross revenues are from government payers like Medicare (the insurance program for persons sixty-five or over and certain other persons under sixty-five with disabilities and end-stage renal disease) and Medicaid (the insurance program for persons with low incomes). Government insurance programs like Medicare and Medicaid pay hospitals less than the cost of treating a patient, so the mix of revenue from government insurance programs and private insurance is critical to the financial health of a hospital. One of Temple Hospital's strategies for increasing the public-private payer mix was to establish specialties like the Lung Center. Temple recruited some of the best pulmonologists and thoracic surgeons in the discipline to form a premiere lung center that attracted patients from outside of the neighborhood and some from out of town, many of them white.

Katie and I went back to the examination room after a short wait in the Lung Center's waiting room. The team had arrived. The two thoracic surgeons, the physician assistant, the nurse, two residents, and several medical students could not have been more accommodating and affirming. They reviewed the plan with compassion and precision. It was a Friday. They scheduled me for preoperative tests three days later on Monday and surgery on Tuesday to remove one-third of my left lung. It would regenerate in about six months. As Katie and I walked back through the waiting room to leave, it was still jammed with patients, many hooked up to oxygen and in wheelchairs. Although I was in this place, I felt out of place. I had no symptoms and no discomfort. I hadn't smoked in nearly twenty years and the spot on my lung was detected on a body scan that was part of a totally unrelated research study on psoriasis. My dermatologist needed participants for his study and I agreed to help out.

The team performed the surgery on Tuesday. The hospital staff couldn't have been more attentive. I quickly connected with the black nurses and other black health-care providers. Our conversations were easy and lighthearted. My brother, a male cousin, and three male friends met up at my single room on day two of a three-day hospital stay. All were pretty good looking. My new nurse friend pretended to come into the room to check something on the contraptions I was hooked up to and whispered in my ear, "There is one handsome guy after another coming in here. You must look different outside of here." Her efforts to make me laugh worked. I was released from the hospital on Friday and back to work ten days later.

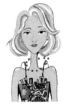 **While Val and I wanted desperately to believe** that her experience was similar to the experience of every patient regardless of race, we knew that it wasn't, particularly for other black patients. There is a deeply disturbing racial component to the provision of health care in the United States. The experiences of racism in education, housing, and employment discussed in Chapter 2 ran alongside racism in health care. Hospitals were segregated, and black patients were relegated to the most underresourced facilities. *The Tuskegee Syphilis Study of Untreated Syphilis in the Male Negro* was one of the most unethical experiments of the U.S. Public Health Service. The forty-year experiment ran from 1932 to 1972 and observed the effects of untreated syphilis on poor and uneducated black men in Alabama. Even after it was determined that syphilis could be treated effectively with penicillin, the antibiotic was intentionally withheld from the participants for decades, leading to death for some and spread of the disease to many of the participants' wives and children.

In 1999, Congress asked the National Academies of Sciences, Engineering, and Medicine, through its Institute of Medicine or IOM (renamed the Health and Medicine Division, or HMD, in 2016) to evaluate racial and ethnic disparities in the quality of health services received by patients in the United States. The 2002 study confirmed that African American patients receive a lower quality of care than their white counterparts when presenting with comparable medical conditions, insurance, income, and age. The conclusions were similar for Latinx patients. The researchers concluded that this health-care disparity is linked to higher death rates among minorities.[2]

For example, black adults presenting to an emergency room generally were triaged to a lower level of care, waited longer for an ICU bed and stroke assessment, and had less chance of being triaged to a coronary care unit.[3] They were less likely to receive even routine medical procedures, be given appropriate cardiac medications, undergo bypass surgery, and receive kidney dialysis or transplants. On the other hand, they were more likely to receive "certain less-desirable procedures," such as amputations for diabetes.[4] And the researchers have confirmed that the disparities were due in part to the biases and prejudices of the health-care providers.

The story is no better for children. Black children who are seen in emergency rooms are less likely than white children to be hospitalized even when they present with similar degrees of abdominal pain, according to a study evaluating health-care outcomes in over four million encounters of abdominal pain in children in the United States. Black children were less likely to get CT scans or surgery than white children for appendicitis which suggests that the scans were not ordered for black children until the condition worsened. Notably, black children had an unexplained 42 percent higher odds of perforated appendicitis, a serious condition leading more often to infection or death.[5]

I take Gabe to doctors for everything from annual checkups with the pediatrician to perhaps an emergency room visit for a minor soccer injury, and the experiences of the vast majority of black children tell me that he will be treated differently and not as well as white children. Assumptions will be made and biases acted upon that will result in Gabe receiving lesser care.

Parents with moderate or significant financial resources may think that because their child has the benefit of a good health insurance plan and access to quality health care, they need not worry about the problems that black children living in communities plagued by poverty and other trauma experience. However, studies tell us that the inferior treatment is often unrelated to income. In fact, low-income white patients received better care—increased odds of hospitalization and imaging for abdominal pain—than high-income black patients.[6] Even as we write this chapter, New York state departments of financial services and health are launching an investigation of racial bias in a commercial health-care algorithm used to identify which patients with complex health needs may benefit from additional resources.[7] Health systems rely on the algorithm to identify patients for specialty programs that provide high levels of care and more attention from health-care professionals. The programs have resulted in improved health outcomes for patients. Using health system records as recently as 2013 to 2015, researchers found that the predictive model for targeting patients with the highest need for the additional resources was constructed using historical data of patients with the highest health-care costs. The bias arises because the algorithm predicts health care costs rather than illness, but unequal access to care means that we spend less money caring for black patients than for white patients.[8] When we talk about a predictive algorithm, think of an occasion where you may go online to purchase something. Amazon, as an example, has made a fortune from using your previous purchases and products you have searched for (your historical data) to predict what future products you may want to purchase. Then their predictive algorithm puts that product conveniently on the screen in front of you. You may wonder, "How does it know?" Now think of over two hundred million historical health records of white and black people who have gained access to medical care. Consider then who received the most extensive and therefore most expensive care among those patients. The predictive formula was built using this data set to target who generated the highest cost of medical care. The researchers' hypothesis was that history would show unequal access to care means that there was less money spent on black people than white people. Not only was this evident in their study, but that algorithm is in play for most health systems across our country.

Val would soon experience the sharp drop-off between a VIP experience of the health-care system and the level of attention and bureaucracy encountered by those who may be less well connected.

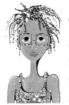 Two and a half years into the annual visits to scan my lungs and check for the possibility of the cancer's recurrence, the dean was moving off the scene. It was much more difficult to get a return call or text and I started raising hell. My daily rantings were tiresome for those around me, including Katie. When I took a breath, Katie very gently suggested, "Just go to another hospital." We had a well-connected colleague who emailed her friend who was a pulmonologist and the director of medicine at a highly-regarded hospital in the city. I received an email inviting me to call his assistant within an hour of him receiving my colleague's email. The same day I got a return call from Temple, there was no need to change hospitals, and I settled down.

However, I really needed to check myself. What had my privilege prompted me to do? I certainly cared about patients who have to wait too long to see a doctor and often can't afford the full range of recommended services and medications. I also empathized with the medical professionals who remain kind, compassionate and giving in the face of limited resources. But I couldn't solve the entire health-care crisis, I reasoned. The reality is I could do something. I could work to expose disparities. I could hear from and advocate for the most marginalized. I could volunteer at the hospital or with organizations working to narrow the gap. Whatever concern I had for others collided with my own self-interest, and self-interest won. I was consumed with how I would fare in all of this. And when I found myself intertwined with others in a health-care system's limitations, instead of offering to be part of a solution that benefitted the whole, I just hollered louder for myself.

The experience also prompted me to consider whether assumptions and biases about race had impacted the health care that people in my family and community had received over the years. Even if not armed with statistics, most black people have enough anecdotal experiences to know that things aren't right. When I was eleven, my mother went to the emergency room of our local hospital on a Thursday evening with excruciating headache pain. She had suffered with scarlet fever as a child. The complications from this "disease of poverty," as it was sometimes called, resulted in a heart murmur. She had a history of hypertension and phlebitis. She was sent home from the emergency room with pain killers. Experiencing no relief, she returned to the emergency room on Friday morning but suffered a cerebral hemorrhage and died on Saturday. She had just turned fifty.

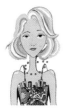 Mike and I know that our presence alone will not ensure that Gabe will not be negatively affected by racial bias. It will take not only my knowledge of the confirmed and yet-to-be confirmed disparities but also knowledge of the unique challenges he faces as a black boy. Sickle cell anemia and sarcoidosis strike black people more than white people, for example. Emerging research suggests that Gabe, Val, and other black people may have a genetic susceptibility to diabetes.

Our first pediatrician for Gabe was a wonderful family friend who, despite nearing retirement, willingly accepted us as her only new patient when Gabe was born. Her decades of practice in an affluent suburban area meant that the majority of her patients were white. While the pediatrician stayed on top of height, weight, head circumference, and the battery of vaccinations, Mike was the one who pressed for blood tests for sickle cell before Gabe turned two. When our beloved pediatrician finally retired when Gabe was seven, we began our search for a black pediatrician. Given our proximity to some of the finest hospitals in the country, we simply could not believe how difficult that was. Even as we started to explore less convenient possibilities, Chad Goller-Sojourner's NPR interview rang in my head. Chad was twenty-five before he saw a black doctor![9]

The fatigue and stress from dealing with it all is enough to make you sick. Whether it's being treated with a lack of appropriate urgency in an emergency room, demeaned in the workplace, relegated to worn-out schools, excluded from opportunities, or suffering physical harm or death at the hands of racist police officers, perceived racial discrimination leads to chronic stress, which is linked to disease and compromised physical health. Specifically, racial discrimination has been associated with a higher risk of breast cancer among black women, particularly younger black women,[10] and higher infant and maternal mortality rates related to the mother's perceived discrimination and resulting stress.[11] As we noted in Chapter 3, experiences of discrimination have been linked to a range of health problems in children, including elevated systolic blood pressure, early onset of insulin resistance depression, attention-deficit/hyperactivity disorder, oppositional defiant disorder, anxiety, and low self-esteem.[12]

Even more, we understand that it's not just the current events like the length of time in a waiting room that can trigger trauma related to racism.[13] Collective trauma from centuries of slavery, legally-mandated discrimination and violent oppression can be passed down through generations even if children do not experience the trauma. And this collective and multigenerational trauma can be triggered today by continued disadvantage, exclusion, discrimination and racial violence toward black people. The result—

disproportionately high rates of depression, anger, stress, hyper-vigilance, and low self-esteem.[14] Because of the effects of collective memory and generational trauma, I recognize that Gabe's reaction to a news report of a black man being shot to death by a white police officer may be different from that of a white boy of similar age. As he, Mike, and I pursue schools, soccer leagues, parishes, and chess clubs, we will do so with the full recognition that as early as now, Gabe will experience the effects of inclusion and exclusion, discrimination and acceptance.

In addition to our knowledge and our awareness, Gabe's well-being also will take our voice. Mike and I will ask questions of health-care providers and insist on answers that we understand. Science also tells us that we must work to provide our children with a good education to ensure their optimal health. Individuals with college degrees generally live longer and have lower rates of chronic disease than those without college degrees.[15] Here is where Mike and I have the great advantage of our white privilege. Our fortune has afforded us the advantage of questioning doctors, nurses, surgeons, and really anyone to whom we have entrusted our health and care. If we were already inclined to do this for ourselves and one another, our inclination has been elevated tenfold to do this for our son. In the upcoming chapters, you will see how Mike and I will continue to use the advantage of our history to the benefit of our family.

6

Not without Education

I tell my students, when you get these jobs that
you have been trained for, just remember that
your real job is that if you are free, you need to
free somebody else. If you have some power, then
your job is to empower somebody else.

—TONI MORRISON

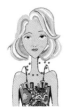 One of the most important and best features of Gabriel's school is its diversity of families and children. Of the eighteen kids who started first grade with him, about two-thirds were students of color. Gabe has been enrolled at this school since before he turned two, and he has never been The Only, ever. This quality has been our deal-breaker when selecting among schools.

When Mike and I purchased our home, we knew that we would be choosing diversity and community, which could mean underfunded public schools. The realtor we were working with even tried to talk us out of our choice. Her instinct was honorable about not buying a house in a neighborhood with low-performing public schools. But our firm desire to put down roots in a house that I fell in love with, and in a community that was different from the all-white neighborhoods where we grew up, tipped the scale. We bought our house in 2003 and had eight long years to contemplate school options before Gabriel was born. Without a child to enroll, we remained loosely aware of what was happening in the school district, and despite how high our taxes felt, they still didn't compare to what our friends were paying in wealthier towns with well-resourced schools. The way that Pennsylvania and most other states finance education divides the haves from the have-nots. State legislators pass most of the burden of financing education to local municipalities, which fund their schools primarily through property taxes. As was more fully discussed in Chapter 2, in the nineteneth century, when public schools in Pennsylvania and their funding scheme were taking shape, wealthy communities—of which black people were rarely a part—had the most resourced schools, while fewer financial resources went to schools in the poorest communities, in which black people were disproportionately overrepresented. In most American states today, public education is still funded through a combination of federal, state, and local resources but relies most heavily on local community resources.

Students of color are often concentrated in schools with fewer resources. Schools with 90 percent or more students of color spend $733 less per student per year than schools with 90 percent or more white students.[1] Today, our majority black neighboring school district is one of six in Pennsylvania petitioning the courts to intervene in the inadequate funding formula. In addition, Pennsylvania is among the ten states contributing the lowest percentage of funding for state education, an allocation already thwarted by this inequitable system.[2] The Philadelphia-based organization Research for Action (RFA)[3] focuses their work on the improvement of educational opportunities and outcomes for traditionally underserved students. RFA's director for policy research, David Lapp, has published several insightful reports on school-, district-, state-, and national-level reform and is preparing a report to show that "Pennsylvania's white students are in the top five of states when it comes to opportunity, including access to such resources as Advanced Placement courses, calculus and physics, dual enrollment with colleges, gifted and talented programs, and disciplinary policies that avoid suspension in favor of restorative justice." Pennsylvania's black students, on the other hand, are in the bottom five of states in terms of access to these opportunities.[4]

As Mike and I neared the time to make a decision about Gabriel's preschool, we went to visit nursery school programs. This was before Gabriel turned two. Strangely, the school I believed would be the whitest turned out to be the most diverse in children and families. Since nursery school would be the first time he would be cared for by nonfamily outside of our home, we also made sure it met other key criteria: warm and nurturing teachers, clean and welcoming classrooms, and 1.5 teachers for seven toddlers. The cafeteria had just baked cookies before we arrived for the tour—genius! Of the seven children in the class, five were children of color. This beautiful palette has persisted every year, with every class since.

When Gabe completed kindergarten, Mike and I were participating for the first time in the official step up ceremony, where preschool through seventh graders gather in the gym on the last day of school, and each class steps up to their new teacher and class line. Parents filed into the humid gymnasium and took their bleacher seats as each class entered the gym in line to take their seat on the hardwood floor. What a sight! The kids were exploding with the joy of being twenty minutes from summer vacation, and their teachers beamed with pride as they prepared to send forth their students to the next venture. Once all the grades were in place, the only class missing was the eighth grade who graduated earlier in the week. The ceremony was marked by each class stepping up and peaks when the seventh graders leap onto the stage at the end of the gym. Class by class, they were announced and cheered on from pre-K to kindergarten, from kindergarten to first, and so on until the seventh graders mount the stage. Admittedly, I filled up with pride as Gabriel's kindergarten class was asked to rise and they took off (five yards) to the first grade line. The whole place went crazy for them, and most of the parents scrambled to capture it all on their smartphones.

Eighteen children—six were white—moved from kindergarten to the next line. The graduating first grade class, seventeen children with a color palette very similar to that of their successors, moved to the second grade line. As second and third grade classes stepped up, the classes were smaller in size and appeared whiter. Each class size gradually became smaller in size until twelve pre-teens excitedly cheered from the stage, two students of color side by side with ten white students. The school could not have presented its difficulty retaining students of color more starkly. My joy turned to confusion even as I sat clapping. Would Gabriel wash out of his class as so many evidently had before him? If not, what would it cost him to remain?

After we got home and celebrated for the rest of the afternoon and evening, we got Gabe to bed, and I returned to the couch to talk with Mike about where that vision of the stepping up ceremony left us. We knew that we wanted to do everything in our power to change that outcome, but I often wondered how and where to start. So I did the thing that helps me organize: I started my email to our new head of school.

Dear Margaret,

As you may know, we have been part of the school community since we enrolled Gabriel in Nursery 2. Since then we have cherished the highs of Kindergarten and the stellar Pre-K year with Mrs. B, and nearly ended our HCA relationship when we were completely disappointed with his Nursery 3 year with a woman who is no longer there.

What you may not be aware of, Mike and I became the highly blessed parents of Gabriel when we matched to him on the day he was born. Observably, Mike and I are the white parents of a mixed-race son. Every day, we work with all our heart to be the best parents, advocates, and guardians of his development and future. This means that we must learn (and unlearn) several things that are different than what our own life journey has taught us.

Perhaps I should have initiated this request and conversation earlier, but here we are. Today, I am better equipped to articulate some of this to you, and as Mike and I have come to see, you are leading and moving our school in ways that we believe resonate for us.

Simply put, we would love for Gabriel to continue here for the next eight years. There are several factors to consider for that to occur, but at the top of the list is maintaining the diversity of his class, which will drive that decision each year. And while it is important to us that the diverse representation among faculty and administrators also grow to mirror the student composition, it is nonnegotiable for our family that Gabriel grows up in an environment that is intentionally designed for his success. This of course means seeing himself as explicitly part of the community of learners.

How we accomplish this together will require work, further education, and seeing ourselves as responsible participants. The consortium of independent schools certainly has extensive guidance for leaders and teachers, but so far my experience with the text, *The Guide for White Women Who Teach Black Boys*,[5] has shown me that there are robust resources for our teachers that will not only support but instruct white adults on the numerous and feasible ways that we can do more in our families, neighborhoods, and schools. I have also found several faculty and administrators who recommend (and even celebrate) the important work of Ali Michael,[6] who coauthored the guide as well as teaches teachers regularly.

Mike and I are not sending this to you without our full commitment to making it happen. Think about ways that we can partner with you, and we would love to meet over the summer to talk and plan.

Congratulations on a wonderful year,
Kate and Mike D'Angelo

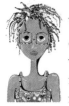 When it comes to their child's education, well-educated white parents are used to being consumers with high expectations—entitled, even. Black parents may be somewhat more measured because they are never quite sure whether the school's subsequent actions are motivated by feelings of resentment toward the parent taken out on the child. And black children will always be more vulnerable to adverse action. Many black parents would worry that a letter such as Katie and Mike composed might backfire. Nonetheless, Katie, Mike, and I share a real concern about the number of black children in Gabe's class and school, as well as the number of black teachers and administrators, because even a well-resourced or elite predominantly white school can leave a black child feeling excluded and isolated, unmotivated, and lacking healthy racial identity. The teachers and administrators at Gabe's school are all white except for the music teacher, who is black.

Having a classroom of children that is so observably different from their teachers is the norm in this country. A report from the U.S. Department of Education looked at racial diversity within the educator workforce in 2011–2012 and found that 10 percent of public school principals were black compared to 80 percent white and that 82 percent of public school teachers identified as white. In addition, black male teachers constituted only 2 percent of the teaching workforce.[7] The stark differences between students and their educators have important effects. Research has shown abundantly that teachers of color can improve the school experiences and academic outcomes for all students, not only for students of color.[8] The evidence shows there are both short-term and long-term positive outcomes if you have a teacher of your same race, including educational attainment and future earnings.[9] Perhaps of greatest importance to some parents, teachers of color are "more likely to confront issues of racism and serve as advocates and cultural brokers" as compared with their peers.[10] It is very clear that a "culturally competent and racially diverse teaching force" is critical if we intend to shape the most effective learning environment for our schools.[11] When 80 percent of teachers are white, and most of their life experience has been formed by Eurocentric history lessons inside of largely segregated communities and schools, it is not a simple pivot for a white teacher to unlearn biases embedded in that narrative.

What can derail black children fast and effectively is the way that white teachers see them. Having and setting low expectations for black children leads to black children being tracked toward less rigorous curriculum and discouraged from pursuing certain professions or opportunities in higher education. There is a growing body of research that has found white teachers have significantly lower educational expectations for black students than do black teachers.[12] Conversely, the positive outcomes of black teachers for black students abound.[13] Specifically, findings revealed that if a black student had just one black teacher by third grade, the student is 13 percent more likely to enroll in college than one who has not, and black students who had two black teachers were 32 percent more likely.[14] One of the reasons: teachers of color tend to set and model higher expectations for students of color.

Katie was on guard toward the expectations her child's school exhibited for Gabe.

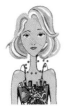 Mike and I are hypersensitive to the notion that anyone would have low expectations for Gabe, particularly the six white women who have been Gabe's teachers since he began preschool. In fact, it was a major contributor when we planned to leave his school when he was four. There is no question from our experience that teachers' expectations influence students' beliefs about their capabilities. As Mike walked Gabe into school on the second to last day

of Nursery 3, he was greeted warmly by the principal on Mike's way out the door. The principal went on to add, "And it really will be good that Gabe will repeat Nursery 3 next year." If it seems like you missed a big chunk of the story that would lead up to that comment, so did we.

Mike made laser eye contact and asked, "What did you just say?"

Had I been in the principal's shoes that morning, I am pretty certain that my context clues would assemble as hers did when she replied, "Mrs. C didn't discuss this with you before going out on leave?"

Mike returned, "Not even a hint."

It took several days to clear the fury we felt from the total lack of communication to outright neglect on the part of Mrs. C, who was responsible for our son for eight months and never thought to mention this possible outcome. As the white mother of a black four-year-old, I can freely tell you that this decision about my black son, made by two white women, set me ablaze. No matter what metrics or rationale the principal was preparing to give us for their decision, we were not on board. Mike and I were not totally clear on how to best advocate for our son, but the plan was to figure it out. The abbreviated version included months of communication with the school and soliciting advice from teachers outside the school and other parents. We learned that Mrs. C would not be returning to the school. We also had the gift of knowing the woman who would be his eventual pre-K teacher, Mrs. B. Because of our trust and confidence in Mrs. B, Mike and I decided to have Gabe start pre-K that September with his class and not repeat Nursery 3. However, once Mrs. B had the opportunity to get to know Gabe, provided daily emails to us with insights and reflections, and met with us outside the classroom, we all agreed by October that transitioning back to Nursery 3 would be the optimal choice for Gabe.

Having that extra time before pre-K was observably meaningful for him. With a September birthday, he went from being the youngest in his class to the oldest. The difference in maturity from age four to five may not seem like a big difference, but I noticed that Gabe's voice sounded clearer, his back stood straighter, and his confidence beamed brighter. It was a full year later when I finally began to exhale, believing that we had advocated for the best outcome. The truth is we may not ever fully know answers before they are in the rearview mirror. In this case, it was months of anger, worry, analysis, relentless engagement, and diligent parenting before we felt sure that we could trust the process again. We were concerned about white teachers having lower expectations for Gabe, and a second area of grave concern to us was that Gabe's behavior would be misperceived.

Behavior of white children that is seen simply as rambunctious and excitable is often perceived in black children as unruly or threatening, resulting in more time spent out of school for discipline that disrupts the education process. Black students are disproportionately disciplined as compared with their white peers. Specifically, black students are three times more likely to be suspended and expelled as white students, according to U.S. Department of Education data. More out-of-school suspensions and expulsions mean they are not in the classroom receiving instruction and other educational support services.[15] Black students are also more than three times as likely to receive one or more out-of-school suspensions as white students for the same behavior.[16] Black girls are especially targeted for discipline. Black girls are suspended at a higher rate (12 percent) than girls of any other race or ethnicity and most boys.[17] Parents of black children must be particularly suspect of punishments for behaviors not defined in the school's code of conduct, like "having an attitude." There are so many things going on in the body and mind of an adolescent girl that these authors don't think we've ever seen a girl with a consistently even attitude. We were prone to have attitudes at that age. However, an attitude may not be perceived the same way in white and black girls. In fact, there is a growing body of research to show that young women of color are particularly subject to push-out practices that contribute to students dropping out of school, including an overreliance on punitive discipline.[18] The research also shows students who are pushed out enter pathways to incarceration at alarming rates.[19]

Education experts agree that removing a student from school should always be the last resort, and policymakers and practitioners recognize that exclusionary disciplinary practices do not improve the quality of children's educational experiences.[20] While the threat of retaliation is always there, the better decision is for parents who believe that their child is being inappropriately targeted to nonetheless be proactive to ensure that appropriate interventions are in place within the school. Request that school administrators document any discipline and send emails or written records of conversations among the student, parents, and administrators. Advocate for the implementation of positive behavior support rather than exclusionary discipline. And if these options are not working, find an education lawyer who focuses on discrimination in education.

An excellent resource for parents, educators, and anyone concerned about creating nurturing learning environments for black children is *The Guide for White Women Who Teach Black Boys*.[21] Scholars, parents, teachers, and student voices, including those of black men and women, are represented by over thirty contributing authors to this extraordinary book. In my roles of parent, educator, coach, colleague, and engaged citizen, I have found *The Guide* to be an extraordinary book that will meet you where you are. As a parent, I tend to be hardwired for determining whether or not the teacher has capacity for making and fostering a positive relationship and nurturing learning environment for our child. "If the teacher does not connect with a student, it is not the fault of the student."[22] The fundamental key to every student's academic success can be tied to an authentically positive relationship to the teacher.

Parents must assess whether the school environment is structured for students' success and whether the institution views black children in a positive way. They should look out for several signs that the school is affirmatively committed to fostering well-being for black students.

1. Is part of the curriculum devoted to understanding African and African American history in a way that dispels false and distorted images and stereotypes?
2. Are black cultural traditions recognized and celebrated?
3. Does your child's book list include works that empower all students, or are stories presented out of context in a way that reinforces notions of inferiority and superiority (you may want to refer back to Chapter 3 for a fuller discussion of the impact of negative images in books and other forms of media)?
4. Is implicit bias training provided for teachers and administrators?
5. Are there recruiting policies and practices in place that encourage diversity among the staff and student body?
6. Has the school implemented alternatives to out-of-school suspensions and incarceration for nonviolent behavior?

As your child moves into high school and SATs, APs, and ACTs become more meaningful, look out for evidence of stereotype threat. When members of a group have been negatively stereotyped, the fear of being judged in light of that stereotype can undermine performance in a given situation. Here's why. Black people, for example, have been stereotyped as less capable intellectually. Black students in a predominantly white school may feel pressure that white students do not experience to dispel the stereotype of intellectual inferiority. The extra pressure to succeed can be a distraction, deplete the student's memory, or require energy to suppress negative thoughts, which means that less of the student's energy and effort can be focused on the task.[23] In at least one small qualitative study, researchers found evidence of the operation of stereotype threat in children as young as seven years old.[24] While the focus of our discussion is race, stereotype threat is not limited to race. Stereotype threat has been found to negatively affect the memory performance of older adults, the math performance of girls, and the performance of white men in sports. Stereotype threats are estimated to account for much of the gender and race gap on the SAT. However, in laboratory tests, when the threat was removed, black students scored equal to white students on SATs, and women performed equal to men on math tests.[25] Outside of the lab, researchers believe reducing the threat will likewise improve performance.[26] Here are a few recommendations for reducing stereotype threats.

1. Educate your child about stereotype threats and help them to recognize the threats as the source of their anxiety.
2. Help your child to understand that the stereotypes are illegitimate.
3. Teach your child to use self-affirmations to reduce the anxiety and refocus.
4. Expose your child to black or female role models of successful performance in the particular area.
5. When the time comes, include some of the roughly one hundred historically black colleges and universities (HBCUs) among the stops on your college tour.

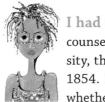 I had the great privilege of serving as general counsel and then as acting president of Lincoln University, the oldest degree-granting HBCU, established in 1854. Because of that experience, I am often asked whether HBCUs are any longer relevant or necessary. HBCUs are defined as "degree-granting institutions established prior to 1964 with the principal mission of educating black Amer-

icans."[27] The argument has been made that HBCUs were established during a time when black people were denied access to predominantly white institutions. Many young people are not impressed when I point to Thurgood Marshall, Langston Hughes, Kwame Nkrumah, and Nnamdi Azikewe as Lincoln graduates; in fact, with the exception of Langston Hughes, most students don't know who the other three are. When I tell them that during the first one hundred years of the existence of HBCUs, they produced the majority of black physicians and attorneys, people ask how that data is meaningful today. They point out that only 9 percent of black students attend HBCUs.[28]

In the 1960s, when black students were provided with greater access and began attending predominantly white institutions in greater numbers, HBCUs suffered in terms of enrollment. In the late 1980s and throughout much of the 1990s, there was a revival of support for HBCUs reflected in films like Spike Lee's *School Daze*. Perhaps that was due to a realization that predominantly white institutions were causing black students some degree of psychological trauma and miseducation. But by the late 1990s and early 2000s, enrollment in HBCUs began to decline again.[29]

I'd like to make the case for consideration of HBCUs for black children. HBCUs are still producing significant numbers of bachelor's degrees for African Americans, particularly in the science, technology, engineering, and math (STEM) fields. While the majority of African American students are not attending HBCUs, if we look at STEM, HBCUs remain a significant producer of bachelor's degrees for African American students in engineering, math, and the sciences. According to a recent United Negro College Fund report, HBCUs produced 25 percent of African American graduates with STEM degrees and 46 percent of black women who earned STEM degrees between 1995 and 2004.[30] Almost 30 percent of black students who have earned a doctorate in science and engineering went to an HBCU as an undergraduate.[31] Might black students in predominately white institutions be getting a message that science isn't for them, a message they are not getting at an HBCU?

As a practical matter, anyone can prepare your child to do a task or get a job. However, many HBCUs do much more. They offer a supportive educational environment for black students, where they see themselves positively. These institutions make it their business to know and share with others an accurate African history—of great African civilizations and leadership and limitless potential. They reinforce the notion that black people are capable of developing ideas, systems, and solutions to advance their own interests. They see the student's potential even when the student doesn't see it. They see the student as valuable, special, and important. Black children live and learn in a space where black leadership and achievement is normative, and where the development of cultural esteem is intentional—which we know leads to achievement. They produce people whose priority is collective responsibility, social consciousness, critical thinking, and the advancement of healthy communities for everyone. In the final analysis, these institutions launch into the world global citizens who believe that education is not solely for individual achievement but is most meaningful when individual achievement translates into progress for everyone. As I presided over the commencement exercise at Lincoln in 2015, the graduate student speaker summed up the value of her HBCU experience. Quoting Langston Hughes, she said, "When people care for you and cry for you, they can straighten out your soul." She concluded her remarks by saying, "Lincoln, thank you for straightening out my soul."

Now as the diversity officer for Temple University, a predominantly white institution (PWI), I am also asked whether the college experience for a black child at a PWI can be culturally relevant and affirming in a way that builds cultural esteem and fosters achievement. My answer is yes. For years, Temple was referred to as "the diversity university," boasting a black student population that exceeded their representation in the general population. Black people are roughly 12 percent of the U.S. population, and a little more than 13 percent of Temple's incoming undergraduate class for the 2019–2020 academic year identify as black. Almost 39 percent of the class identify as persons of color. Today, black Temple students tag their robust community "Black Temple." The university is proud to have one of the country's finest African American Studies departments, whose graduates include actor Jesse Williams and two of this generation's most recognized and highly regarded academic thought leaders, Eddie Glaude Jr. and Ibram X. Kendi and which is chaired by leading Africology scholar Molefi K. Asante. More than thirty years ago, the department began offering the world's first Ph.D. in African American Studies, and it has since graduated almost two hundred doctoral candidates who now engage in a range of activities, including serving as chairs of African American Studies departments at institutions across the country. I point to Temple as an example of an institution that has been intentional about creating a space that is inclusive and welcoming to black students. Do a little research to determine the extent to which the institutions your child is considering demonstrate that commitment. University websites may contain demographic information, including the number of black students, faculty, and staff, and if there is an institutional diversity office it can be an excellent source of information regarding the institution's diversity efforts.

If your child has school, family, or community networks that include other black people, they may easily navigate black spaces and, once on campus, will immediately begin to make connections and create pathways to diverse social experiences. A college campus can present an exciting opportunity for a black child who has been raised with few connections to black culture or community to make these connections as well. However, it is not uncommon for black children to initially be rejected by their black peers if they lack cultural commonalities, whether it be language, experiences, music preferences, or swagger. Connections are still possible, however. It will simply take a more intentional effort.

Encourage them to join organizations engaged in activities of interest to black students and to which black students generally belong, like the Black Student Union, the student divisions of black professional organizations like the National Association of Black Engineers, or black Greek-letter fraternities and sororities. Most school websites include a list of student organizations, and most schools have an organization fair at the beginning of the fall semester.

Recommend that they take classes in the school's African American Studies department and consider a major or minor in the discipline.

Advise them to connect with the university's institutional diversity office or center. These offices generally sponsor programs and events of interest to students of color and create opportunities to meet a diverse group of students. Students get a great benefit from hanging out at the office, attending programs, and volunteering for service opportunities.

Suggest that they engage in activities that give them exposure and respect, like giving campus tours, applying to be a resident assistant, volunteering for service projects, and participating in leadership development programs.

Above all, tell them to be persistent about getting what they came for: new and diverse experiences!

In most circles we travel, we consistently hear that education is the "great equalizer." However, passive education environments equalize nothing for black children. There is a critical role for parents to make sure the learning environment is constantly examined and intentionally designed to achieve positive educational outcomes for children of all races and backgrounds. But it goes far beyond whether your child knows the fundamentals of multiplication, memorizes the periodic table of elements, or can speak three languages, all of which helps, even if it's insufficient. For black students, the rate of referrals to law enforcement (27 percent) and school-related arrests (31 percent) exceed their representation in the student body (16 percent). White students, on the other hand, comprise 51 percent of the study body but only 41 percent of the law enforcement referrals and 39 percent of arrests.[32] These numbers are important because there is a demonstrable link between what happens in school and subsequent incarceration, commonly referred to as the school-to-prison pipeline. In Chapter 7, we will share some resources parents can use in an effort to keep their children safe.

7

The Talk

I figured I'd have to explain some name-calling,
have hard talks about language, navigate the waters
when somebody's parent won't let my son take their
daughter to prom . . . At no point did I think I would
have to teach my son how to stay alive.

—KAREN VALBY[1]

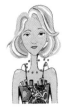 Many Americans clung to the hope that Trayvon Martin's death was an explainable, isolated incident. In my limited view and experience, I could have been inclined to believe that clear reasoning would emerge. Details would be revealed to make us resume our comfort and confidence in the system in place to protect us. Surely, I would wait it out and the justification would unfold. But then Michael Brown. But then Eric Garner. And then twelve-year-old Tamir Rice. Walter Scott, Freddie Gray, the Charleston Nine, Aiyana Jones, Philando Castile—the news just kept coming, the facts of each case compounding my new reality. The comfort and confidence I had been clinging to had been constructed to secure me and others like me. The description of each stolen life matched the color of my son in this unrelenting cascade.

One does not have to look far in the news or recent events to know that black men and women of all ages are confronted with unconscionable violence simply for being black. Whether it's the high school student required to cut his dreadlocks or forfeit his wrestling match, or a twelve-year-old playing alone in a park with a pellet gun who was shot and killed by a police officer, the enforcement apparatus prioritizes the punishment of black bodies that threaten white spaces. That apparatus—police, the education system, the housing system, zoning and tax policy—prioritizes the security of white people in comfort and confidence, as it has since it was built. Our focus here will not only share advice gleaned from experts that parents can use but will also unveil the unreformed systems that we must all work to change for our village.

If you have ever been a parent or loved another person more than yourself, you should understand the difficulty of grappling with the reality of threats to your child. It is our human instinct to hear about a tragic event and identify the cause so we can rule it out for ourselves. Someone is diagnosed with lung cancer—they smoked, I don't, I'm good. Tornadoes tear a town apart—it happened in Kansas, it's called tornado alley for a reason, I live in Philly, I'm good. Someone is shot and killed holding a cell phone in his grandmother's backyard in Sacramento, in his own apartment in Dallas, for a broken taillight, for selling a loosie on the street—what are you ruling out?

As white parents of a brown child, we are becoming keenly aware of the behaviors, attitudes, whims, and words we've been afforded with the privilege of our race. Our privilege has allowed us to break curfews, drive fast, question authority, and remain unfazed by the consequences. When I think back to the night we arrived at the hospital where Gabriel was born, it was our sheer will that propelled us to the security desk expecting to see a newborn that we did not yet have a shred of legal relationship to meet. There have been plenty of occasions when Mike and I have challenged doctors, lawyers, police officers, priests, and supervisors and questioned their judgments or decisions. We've had to understand that our decisions and behaviors that others read as assertive could be read as disorderly, defiant, or even threatening if we were not white. Our world does not give our son the privilege of acting like us, and moreover, it places on him the burden of managing how others feel about him.

When Gabriel was seven, the three of us were riding home together late in the evening after having dinner with friends. For no particular reason, an older white man in a minivan decided to make some antagonizing moves and cut into our lane.

Mike is not what I would call a defensive driver. He is, in fact, an aggressive driver. I would add this to the list of behaviors and attitudes that our privilege has afforded us. Mike accelerated. Old white guy slowed ahead of us so we wouldn't make the light. Mike accelerated around old white guy, illegally into the opposite lane. Old white guy floored it to block Mike from turning onto our exit and then stopped. Mike likely wanted to drive his truck up and over the guy and his minivan but swerved around and past him.

My blood boiled, and I snapped. "Knock it off! Drive like you care about the other people in this truck!" My fury only enraged Mike more.

The tandem of angry white men jockeyed for position, and my mind raced ahead to how quickly this scene could implode. I desperately wanted to go off on Mike, but we had committed to never diminishing one another in front of Gabriel. While it was not unusual for me to be annoyed by Mike's driving, this was more than simple aggravation. My skin was prickling and burning now as I swallowed back everything I wanted to unleash.

The old white guy rolled off in another direction, and we continued home, barreling down the highway. Gabriel tossed in some commentary from the booster seat behind us, but most of it was lost on me. I couldn't hear anything because I was lost in my own scenario plotting. The next thing I did hear was Mike. I can't remember his exact words or their order, but what registered in my brain was some combination of "Don't ever yell at me like that again."

At that point, a bolt of rage flashed through me, and in a low voice, I lunged, "You arrogant, privileged white boy. Don't you ever model behavior that would get our child killed."

We eventually got home, and the stone silence remained throughout the night and into morning. Perhaps the most import-

ant part of this story is that the next morning, Mike asked Gabriel and me if he could speak to both of us about last night. He sat
us down and said, "I'm sorry." The timing of this book in the life of
our parenting experience is such that we are learning in real time.
When Mike and I examine our history and who communicated key
lessons to us and prepared us for moments and milestones, our
race didn't appear to us to inform any of it. If we indulged our road
rage, trespassed as kids, tried a joint, took a better seat at a stadi-
um, or mouthed off to a stranger for cutting in line, our whiteness
allowed our action to be seen as the normal testing of boundaries
or the temporary neediness of an emotional being in society, not
as a criminal danger to law and order, showcasing the heart of who
we are. It is only now that we understand how very different it all
was for us because of the color of our skin. Our friends who are
black have had a lifetime of feedback about how their actions
might be perceived as threats and how different communities have
managed that experience.

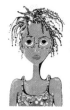 As a child in one of Philadelphia's all-black pub-
lic elementary schools in the late 1960s and early
1970s, my brother, my schoolmates, and I were period-
ically ushered into the auditorium for a special assem-
bly. Black police officers would remind us to be respect-
ful of authority. It was not uncommon for the officer to be familiar
to us. He (female officers were not admitted to the Philadelphia
police academy until 1976) may have lived on our street or was a
regular in the neighborhood barbershop. This was long before the
Internet and before our parents' guidance was identified by the
moniker "the talk." Brutality against black people at the hands of
law enforcement is as old as the history of black people in the United States, and the instructions and advice of black elders have
always gone hand in hand with that reality. "Walk like you have
somewhere to go," they'd tell us. While there were no guarantees,

they gave us their best advice to increase the chances that we would escape the criminal justice system and stay alive.

While every generation of black Americans has been aware of the danger they face from authorities and shared strategies to avoid conflict, the indignity and uncertainty of a fundamentally skewed lottery has also inspired a steady flow of resistance, and from time to time that resistance grows to the point that it prompts a reactionary blowback that places black communities in further danger still.

Organizations like the Black Panther Party—armed with a keen knowledge of their legal rights and a determination to disrupt life as Americans had known it—wanted to remedy those things that guaranteed that white families had the opportunities to enjoy privilege and advancement while black families disproportionately remained locked in poverty or advanced at an anemic pace: unequal education, housing and employment discrimination, inadequate health care.

In the late 1960s the party was headquartered in Northern California, and members brandished their weapons in the face of police on the streets of Oakland. Party leader Huey Newton, who was an avid student of the law and actually attended San Francisco Law School, knew that California state law allowed people to carry guns as long as they were not concealed. In 1967, the Oakland group began to openly arm themselves and monitor the police. When members of the group were confronted by police, they boldly recited portions of the constitution that established their right to carry guns.[2] The Black Panthers also marched into the California state capitol in Sacramento and entered the floor of the legislature during a debate to protest a bill that would limit the right of California citizens to carry loaded weapons.[3]

Branches were organized in major cities throughout the United States, and party members established social programs like breakfast for schoolchildren, child care centers, legal aid services, music classes, GED classes, political education classes, voter registration, and food giveaways. At its height, the party had over ten thousand members, fifty thousand supporters, and thirty-two chapters.[4]

In September 1968, J. Edgar Hoover, then director of the Federal Bureau of Investigations (FBI), "designated the Black Panther Party as the greatest threat to the internal security of the country."[5] Hoover's fears led him to initiate a massive counterinsurgency agenda designed to destroy the party and groups like it, to prevent militant black nationalist groups and leaders from gaining respectability by discrediting them, and to prevent the rise of a messiah who could unify and electrify a movement for equal rights. Published reports indicate that as a result of that effort, "by the end of 1969 it was estimated that 30 Panthers were facing capital punishment, 40 faced life in prison, 55 faced terms up to thirty years, and another 155 were in jail or being sought."[6] The use of wiretaps without judicial approval was rampant, and the FBI specifically directed local law enforcement to "disrupt and neutralize the Black Panther Party."[7]

In 1970, relations between Philadelphia Black Panther members and Philadelphia police commissioner Frank Rizzo came to a head. Rizzo had already gained some degree of infamy for his brutality against black people. In the summer of 1970, there was an attempt made to blow up a police guardhouse, and one police officer was killed and another was injured. In a separate incident the next day, two officers were shot but survived. Although there was little evidence to support the suspicion that the Black Panthers were involved in the incidents, Rizzo nonetheless declared on a local radio show, "Every black revolutionary would be locked up by sun up."[8] And Rizzo embarked on a mission to do just that. At the end of the day, Rizzo had raided three Black Panther office locations and ransacked, teargassed, and terrorized party members in their offices. At one location, the police marched members out of the office, lined them up against the wall, and unclothed them in an effort to publicly humiliate them in front of the media—whom, by the way, Rizzo had invited to witness the raids. The local story was picked up by the national press.[9] Rizzo gloated, "Imagine the big Black Panthers with their pants down!" Fourteen Panthers were arrested, and three police officers were injured.[10] I recall my mother's outrage at the cover picture of these stripped men forced to submit to unfounded police actions and the thick air of resentment that flowed through our black neighborhood after.

The Philadelphia party was to some degree born out of Rizzo's heavy-handedness. After a group of predominantly black citizens gathered at the Philadelphia Board of Education building in November 1967 seeking improvements in education for the city's public school students, Rizzo ordered police to "get their black asses."[11] Some of the participants in the demonstration were so incensed by the commissioner's actions that they began meeting to discuss the black struggle in Philadelphia.[12] The party's Philadelphia branch formed out of these meetings, and the first official party meeting was in May 1969 on the 1900 block of Columbia Avenue in North Philadelphia, just five blocks from Temple University's campus where Katie and I have worked for decades.

Shortly after the 1970 raid, the Philadelphia chapter hosted the party's September 1970 national conference. Father Paul Washington of North Philadelphia's Church of the Advocate and then Philadelphia Bar Association president Robert Landis helped secure the church and Temple University as the venue for the massive meeting.[13]

In late 1970, the chapter also filed a lawsuit seeking injunctive relief, asking that the Philadelphia Police Department be put into federal receivership and be prevented from further harassment of the party members. The case ultimately resulted in an adverse decision for the party. Rizzo became mayor in 1972 and campaigned on the promise that he would control what he considered the dangerous segments of the black community. He subsequently served for two terms. The tone and tenor of Rizzo's reign informed how policies and protocol would be decided for the "City of Brotherly Love."

While this was before the Internet and social media and during a time when much of the news was confined to the local or regional community, the 1969 raid of the Black Panther party residence in Chicago and the killing of Chicago chapter leader Fred Hampton and Mark Clark could not escape national attention. As a result of the incident, those party members who survived the raid were arrested and criminally prosecuted, there was a coroner's inquest, and the Chicago Police Department undertook an internal investigation of the incident. A federal and two state grand jury investigations were convened, and indictments were issued against a number of the officials, including then Cook County state attorney Edward V. Hanrahan, for conspiring to obstruct justice. Indictments were returned because virtually all of the bullets fired were from police weapons.[14] The defendants were ultimately acquitted, however.

As children, we didn't fully understand all that was going on in Philadelphia and around the country between black people and police, but we knew it was a mess. At the same time, the musical genius of Earth, Wind and Fire and Stevie Wonder; the beauty and majesty of the Afro and the dashiki; pride in the power of Muhammad Ali and Black Olympians with raised fists; and the literary brilliance of Toni Morrison and Ismael Reed coexisted with this violence. Then and now, we learn to live in the tension of the contradictions of cruelty and beauty. And our marching orders are the same: remove any perception that we are a threat to the police. As one officer explained, when you encounter the police, "you have to let them know what they got." That first means the burden is on you, even if you are a child, to reassure an adult officer that you are compliant and will work to deescalate the situation if necessary. Extensive research shows that police consistently treat civilians differently by skin tone. Specifically, black civilians have a 27 percent greater chance of experiencing police use of force during a stop and a 28 percent greater chance of officers drawing their guns when compared with white civilians.[15] Letting them know what they got is imperfect advice that may not always work, but it is a necessary skill.

A decade or so after those grade school assemblies, I began my first year as a law student at Villanova University. The campus is nestled in one of the most exclusive communities in suburban Philadelphia, and the sixteen-mile trek from Philly took me through the region's wealthiest neighborhoods. While my Chevrolet Chevette was no match for the Beamers and Benzes that dominated the road, I cruised along with the pack. Within the first several weeks of beginning law school, white township police officers stopped me repeatedly—for speeding, they said. Knowing that police tend to stop black people more often than white people,[16] I always had my law school textbooks in full view on the passenger side seat to let them know what they got.

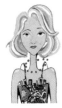

What Val, her brother, and her classmates knew in the 1960s, 1970s, and 1980s continues to be backed up by the research. Black adults are treated more harshly than white adults by the criminal justice system.[17] Black people are still stereotyped as criminal and violent, and they are perceived as less innocent than white people.[18] As we introduced in Chapter 6, black children are often misperceived as older than their years and held accountable for behaviors when "their peers receive the beneficial assumption of childlike innocence."[19] As a result, schools disproportionately impose more out-of-school suspensions and expulsions on black children, particularly black girls, compared with their white classmates, and the criminal justice system often treats them with severity more appropriate for adults by cutting them off from their families, disrupting their education, and even confining them to facilities where they experience more trauma or violence.[20] Not only can these disciplinary measures create emotional and behavioral problems, but there is an established correlation between school discipline and entry into the criminal justice system.[21]

There is not one definitive explanation for why this school-to-prison pipeline exists, however common theories point to lack of supervision during periods of suspension or expulsion, disengagement with the educational process, and acceptance of a perceived role as a troublemaker and as culprits.[22] Other theorists believe the pipeline is fueled by schools' zero tolerance policies.[23] In the mid-1990s, Congress responded to a rash of school shootings by enacting the Gun Free Schools Act of 1994. The law required schools to enforce zero tolerance policies for weapons violations by expelling students or risk losing federal funding. Schools began expanding the range of infractions to include alcohol and drug violations, fighting, dress code violations, and more subjective behaviors like insubordination and disruptions. Or could the school-to-incarceration life course be due to the same issues that disproportionately plague many black children—poverty, abuse, inadequate schools, and all that comes with that—continuing to plague them as adults and limiting or locking them out of legal opportunities to economically sustain themselves and their families.

For a deeper dive into a discussion of the various policies and practices that drive mass incarceration and violence against black people at the hands of law enforcement, consider Michelle Alexander's *The New Jim Crow: Mass Incarceration in the Age of Colorblindness; Locking Up Our Own: Crime and Punishment in Black America* by James Forman Jr. and *Just Mercy* by Bryan Stevenson.

On December 18, 2014, just over four months after a Ferguson, Missouri, police officer fatally shot eighteen-year-old Michael Brown, President Barack Obama signed Executive Order 13684, establishing a President's Task Force on Twenty-First Century Policing.[24] The president charged the task force with "identifying the best means of providing an effective partnership between law enforcement and local communities that reduces crime and increases trust in a country where too many individuals, particularly young people of color, do not feel as if they are being treated fairly."[25] The final task force report calls for police forces to, among other things, create diverse workforces and provide instruction for police officers on explicit bias (the conscious bias we have about certain populations based upon attributes such as race and socioeconomic class) as well as implicit bias (the biases that people are not even aware that they hold).[26] The promising news is that such training has proven to change behavior.[27]

In the meantime, I dread that we need to give our son specific strategies to minimize the risk of an encounter with police going terribly wrong. Again, any strategy comes with imperfections, and there are no guarantees. Our guiding principles remain the same. Mike and I are teaching Gabriel a healthy sense of respect for authority across the board—for teachers, elders in our village, and police charged with serving and protecting him. We will tell him that while not everyone is racist, some people are. We also will tell him that most everyone, including his family that loves him deeply, carries some degree of implicit or unconscious bias. We will tell him that some police officers will be kind and act in his best interest while others will be afraid of him or want to hurt him. You simply don't know what you're going to get.

After combing through media resources, considering arguments both for and against having the talk,[28] and receiving expert advice from a big-city police commissioner, other police officers, and black men and women with firsthand experience, we will tell him if he is stopped by police in a car or on foot:

1. Pull over, roll down the window, and turn on the interior lights (if you are in a car).
2. Make sure your hands are visible at all times.
3. Don't reach for anything or get out of the car unless you are asked to do so by police, and even suggest that the officer reach for your credentials.

4. Do what you're told.
5. Even if you believe you were stopped unjustly or are being treated unfairly, we'll deal with it later. This is not the time to argue.
6. Ask the officer for permission to call your parent; again, don't reach for your phone unless given permission, and even suggest that the officer retrieve it for you.

We also recommend that you read and provide your child with a copy of the *Tamir Rice Safety Handbook*, a short online guide prepared by the ACLU Ohio.[29]

The truth is when I envision scenarios of Gabriel being unfairly disciplined by a teacher, having his symptoms dismissed in an overrun hospital waiting room, or being shadowed in a store by a security guard, each time, I exhale because either Mike or I is with him. What makes any of these scenarios—including ten years from now when he could be driving—so fearful is the common experience of any parent: preparing children for the occasion when you are not there. The principles remain the same whether my son is stopped by a police officer or overlooked by an ER doctor: your one and only job is to come home safe to us. Even if that means that you have been mistreated, insulted, or underestimated, you try as hard as you can to breathe, reduce your fear, and deescalate theirs, and when you get home, we stand ready to do whatever we need to do.

Not only must we have the talk with Gabriel, but we must also have another talk with everyone else around him that has been gifted with never even knowing there was a talk. Here, I echo Maralee Bradley and her poignant letter, "Dear White Parents of My Black Child's Friends: I Need Your Help."[30] Maralee is the mother of six children, and her deeply compassionate plea is to inform her community that no matter how much she does to teach and prepare her own children about racism and injustice, we need our fellow white parents, neighbors, and children's friends to think and change as well.

As painful as it is to accept that my black child is held to a very different standard than his white peers, the parents of white children need to do more than promote colorblindness. And yes, this is as much a call to action for you as anyone. In fact, being born white may be exactly where the phrase "dodged a bullet" originated. If you really want to count yourself progressive, then teach your child about racism and talk to them about what they could do when they see it happening on the playground, in the classroom, or in a retail store. Help your children to interpret unfair treatment and confront it when they can. As soon as it's age appropriate, teach your children how to lift some of the unnecessary burden off the child who cannot make the same mistakes a white child is allowed. Explain thoughtfully and carefully that driving fast, drinking underage, running through other neighbor's yards, sneaking into a private pool after hours, or playing with plastic guns in a park may seem like harmless games that place my black son at risk.

From one parent to another, believe that my fear for my child's life and security is as searing as yours. At the heart of it all, this book intends to reach the ever-growing families that share similar experiences and stories and bring them into a community of support. This chapter cannot simply lay out suggestions for parents of black children because we can no longer make the child responsible for the adults. Perhaps one day, we will all have a new variation on the talk, and it will include more people in the conversation than just my son and a future police officer. At this point in the book, we should safely assume that you have bought in and wholly get that the apparatus will be changed only when white parents and their families also use the tools in their toolkit.

8

Alchemy of Intention

Shallow understanding from people of good will is
more frustrating than absolute misunderstanding
from people of ill will. Lukewarm acceptance is
much more bewildering than outright rejection.
—REVEREND DR. MARTIN LUTHER KING JR.

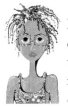 Becoming our best selves, fully human, is an
evolutionary process that requires hard changes. Along
the journey, we often slip in and out of bad decision making and misguided activism. In terms of racial equity, we
can embrace ideas and behaviors that on their face may
appear righteous but in reality thwart the cause, like white fragility,
colorblindness, postracialism, and even philanthropy. The more
insidious culprit is a self-interest that fails to recognize the perspectives and interests of others as equal to our own. Katie and I know
all too well that engaging in an introspective process to discover our
blind spots, calling them out, and then doing something about them
(changing our behavior) takes a level of courage. It is our sincere
hope that sharing our story of self-discovery will make it easier for
you to explore and share these ideas in your own lives.

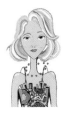 Another value that we treasure about Gabe's
school is the focus on community and connectedness
among the families. There were three children from
Gabe's kindergarten class that did not continue to first
grade at the school. All three children were African

American. Three new children filled their seats, and the three new children also happened to be African American. From the moment we knew the families enrolled, Mike, Gabe, and I committed to welcoming them to the community and making them feel part of our class. When an e-invitation to one of the new boy's birthday parties arrived in my inbox, I hardly consulted the calendar before promptly responding yes.

On the day of the party, the three of us drove the thirty-six miles to a neighboring state and arrived six minutes early. The place was pretty much a hub of overstimulation with an arcade on steroids, a full bowling alley, a ropes course of daredevils traversing over our heads, and a full-blown sports bar with screens of action spanning every wall. The whole scene, while not my cup of tea, sent an instant jolt of joy and energy through every cell in Gabe's little body. The place was straight up mobbed with people and partially organized chaos.

I maneuvered toward a seventy-two-inch plasma screen with what appeared to be party and group assignments. I spotted the name of the birthday boy attached to a time that was thirty minutes earlier than the invitation had instructed us to arrive. With that, I approached the host station to announce our arrival and find out where to go. The nice young woman replied, "The family has not arrived yet, but we can get your child's size for bowling shoes."

I gave her Gabe's shoe size and then caught the attention of another dad and classmate who had similarly arrived early. As I told Val this story, she correctly suspected that this other early arriver was also white. As Gabe and his friend inspected the waiting area and peered out into the sea of madness in store for them, I made small talk with Mike and the other dad while judgmentally recalling the setup and decorating I do early for my son's parties. The two o'clock hour came and went, and more families from school trickled into the waiting area. Mike called the number on the party invitation to find out where the missing party family could be, and the response he got at 2:15 was, "We're pulling up now." Ten more minutes pass, and the birthday boy arrived with his parents and some additional family in tow. Mike, the other early dad, and I were the only white adults at the party. My impatience was tempered somewhat, but not completely, when I recalled that my sense of time was connected to my worldview, and their worldview was equally logical and actually common in other spaces.

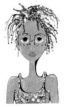 African Americans often evidence a mysterious collective memory, a retention of African practices and behaviors that we may not have been explicitly taught but that we nonetheless exhibit. One afternoon, I was kicking back with two black Temple Africology students, and the three of us marveled at the phenomenon. "Africans traditionally didn't have a notion of the future in the same sense as Western philosophy," Taharka Adé explained. Taharka is a doctoral student whose research is focused on precolonial African paradigms. His speech is unhurried and eloquent with a hint of a Southern accent evidencing his Alabama roots. "In traditional African societies, we did not have a strict concept of time. The African's plan was based on what was necessary to move in the present. Past and present were inseparable. An African worldview is guided by notions of continuation and not concepts of time. We live on in our children, in our community. The African notion is of longevity and rebirth through the ancestral plane."

"Disney has branded it in the African tale *The Lion King*—Hakuna Matata, no worries," his wife, Imani, chimed in.

On the other hand, "Western philosophy is connected to eminence, so we have to be on top of our game. We are obsessed with moving forward, consumed with development. Our ethos is individualism. Because time is considered finite for many Americans, we can't waste it," Taharka concluded as I stood up, defying the collective memory to rush to the next thing on my crowded agenda.

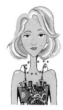 **Once the birthday boy and his family arrived** and greeted the waiting guests, we all filed back to the reserved bowling lanes, and the kids proceeded to have a ball. While they were happily occupied, I had an opportunity to talk to a couple of the parents, including the mom of the other new boy to the class. I felt like we immediately clicked. She is an African American woman who grew up in Philly and graduated from schools that Mike and I know well. Her son is an only child, and the bond we shared of raising a boy made the conversation flow effortlessly.

After an hour of bowling and pizza, I was exceedingly ready for cake and the hour drive home. The young lady assigned to manage our group announced to the kids it was time to line up so we could proceed over to play laser tag. A few items flooded my brain: (1) We don't allow guns or games involving guns, so this announcement pissed me off. (2) Gabe is beaming because of this, and he smartly intuits that I will not make a scene and pull out (Dada might, but not Mama). (3) We started this party a full thirty minutes late because of the host family's tardiness, so why is this event not over?

Gabe's excitement won, and all of us followed the line of children to the other side of this behemoth to the laser tag zone. The line of twenty kids was single file because one at a time, they were being publicly measured by the height requirement on the wall.

My stomach started doing violent backflips because I knew Gabe would not make the forty-eight-inch mark. Somehow, he also anticipated this highly visible failure, and I could see his embarrassment reddening his cheeks. Birthday boy's father and two buddies cruised through, as did the other fifteen boys at the party. Gabe was the only boy who was denied.

If emotions could govern that moment, Mike would have unleashed on the place, and I would have been right there with him. Birthday boy's dad and two buddies were black and said absolutely nothing. Birthday boy's mom and their family and friends were all black and turned their attention somewhere other than where I needed them. All the other parents and children were black, as were the two employees enforcing the height requirement and the manager who was eventually summoned.

Split-second decisions are necessary in such moments, and I saw the employee hand Gabe an arcade card to go play while all the other boys went on to laser tag. I grabbed him and, with the fakest smile I could conjure, said, "Let's go play anything you want."

Every fiber of Mike and me wanted to tear apart that place and every adult responsible. I desperately needed Gabe to rebound and headed straight for some game that I would never let him so much as look at. But that didn't happen. He was crushed.

It's only through a lot of reflection and conversation with Val that I've been able to put a finger on why I was so bothered and frustrated with myself at the time and sort out whether or not I'd done the right thing.

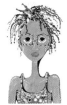 The black fathers at the birthday party probably did not intervene because Gabe did not meet the height requirement and therefore was not entitled to partici-pate in that particular game. They probably expected that Gabe would be happily redirected to alternative activities. Katie's feelings in the moment presented a red flag for Katie and me as we wondered whether her response was motivated or hindered by race in some way. While Katie's instinct to stand up for Gabe and bend the rules to protect him comes from a place of care—and indeed, an appropriate sensitivity to how the world might treat him differently—it doesn't necessarily set Gabe up for success. Gabe will need to develop a certain resilience. Were he to expect every slight to be worthy of making a scene and calling a manager, he would end up exhausted from the emotional labor and burden of trying to bring about a fairer world single-handedly—and so would Katie. One might question whether this parental instinct

even serves the long-term mental health of white children, who may encounter fewer slights in white spaces than their peers of color but are certainly not immune from embarrassment or disappointment and need to develop resilience and discretion in their encounters with authority as well. Certainly, all parents want to protect their children from discomfort. However, Gabe will have to regularly endure a range of discomforting situations because of the actions of racist individuals and the operation of racist policies. The often daily indignities, called microaggressions by some, will range from questions like "Why do you talk white?" to the guaranteed encounter with a white woman who will clutch her purse or lock her car at the sight of him. It also may mean looking down the barrel of the gun of a racist police officer. And in each case, although he is a child, he will be responsible for making the adult feel comfortable and getting out of the situation intact because he can never be sure he will receive the same consideration that his white peers would have received. Gabe will need to become skilled at regularly distinguishing between legitimate authority and racist actions, as will Katie, and to appropriately respond in a way that does not leave him depleted but strong in character and resilience, accountable and responsible. Entitled thinking limits these growth opportunities for any child but could also be dangerous for a black child who has to navigate a racist society. Katie understandably feels very anxious about preparing Gabe for experiences she has never known and fears that her insulation will misguide him as he faces the challenges ahead. The events at the birthday party continued to reveal some of this in small doses.

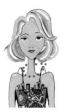 As we began to retreat to the hundreds of alternative activities at the party, out of nowhere came the mom I was bonding with just minutes before. For reasons you will soon understand, I will now refer to her as SuperMom. SuperMom slid her hand into Gabe's,

and they jogged hand in hand back to the laser tag zone, where our group was listening to a safety video and putting on vests to play. She nudged Gabe into the mix and started to help him put a vest on and buckle it. The two employees called for managerial backup, and one such manager, an older black gentleman, appeared. Super-Mom moved straight to him, and I stayed close on her hip, though she clearly did not need anyone.

Calmly and discretely, SuperMom laid it all out with a clarity and poise I not only appreciated but envied. "It is unfortunate that this activity and the requirements to play were not made clear to us ahead of time, but here we are. When there are fifteen boys and only one cannot participate because of an inch, then accommodations need to be made."

Now, it is quite likely that everyone assumed that SuperMom was Gabe's mother. If that was what got the manager to acquiesce, I am good with it. Gabe rejoined the party, and for the next twenty minutes, he was in his own little heaven. All Mike and I could muster were a hundred thank-yous. When it was time to go home, I reminded Gabe to thank SuperMom because had it not been for her voice, he would not have had the opportunity. In addition to preventing Gabe from feeling excluded, the mother's other motivation was probably to make the white parents feel comfortable and not have them feel alone. Because we're not used to feeling excluded, she wanted to spare others that pain and take care of people she viewed as vulnerable in that moment. She took on the burden of advocacy so that Gabe, Mike, and I didn't have to or wonder whether we ought to have.

Dr. Beverly Daniel Tatum's highly acclaimed book *Why Are All the Black Kids Sitting Together in the Cafeteria?* is among the many texts that we hope you will seek out on your parenting journey. Dr. Tatum spends a chapter acknowledging the paralysis of fear, particularly as it relates to white people feeling immobilized by the fear of speaking about race and racism.[1] This is meaningful for me because it helps to give me words to describe the self-imposed constraints I placed on myself when I chose not to confront my son's exclusion from an activity. Some may read my version of the birthday party and missing a height requirement as over-the-top or entitled. Others may wonder why I was unnecessarily stifled and didn't step up to the manager on my own and use my voice. All fair ponderings. Dr. Tatum and her interviewees articulated the undercurrent of my fear for me. While I am not generally a person that shies from confrontation, I am when I perceive that I am in the experiential minority. As the only white woman in the room, I was most afraid of being seen as privileged, arrogant, and offensive; therefore, provoking a negative response from the family (we were their invited guests) or the managers that could be embarrassing or create even more disruption than my son's denial.

This fear of using my voice was such a rare instance for me that I couldn't identify what was really at work. As I thought about it further, I concluded that what was at work was rooted in fear and framed by the color of my skin (when compared to others). I began to appreciate more how incredibly comfortable and confident I am when I am not the minority in the room—which was everywhere else but this party. Pick this party up and put it in a white space, with a white manager and a white father of the birthday boy, and it probably would never have made it to this book. Instead, my silence felt deafening. I revel in the occasions where I have made a sport of inviting conflict, sparring with bosses over a decision and openly disagreeing with a dominant opinion. This moment showed me the freedom that an absence of fear affords me in those spaces. And it leaves me pained because I realize how crippling the fear might be for the black or brown voice. Moreover, just as I was ready to relate the facility's enforcement of its rules to my awareness of race in that moment, I found myself experiencing a defensiveness akin to that felt by many black people in white spaces who might be quick to wonder whether their race had affected their treatment and whether I shouldn't raise the issue just to make sure I wasn't being taken advantage of. But my ability to navigate this distinction was hampered by my newness to this awkward position. It became clear that much of my perspective is acutely influenced by my white fragility, a term coined by Robin DiAngelo, and that is a blind spot for many white people:

> Given how seldom [white people] experience racial discomfort in a society we dominate, we haven't had to build our racial stamina. Socialized into a deeply internalized sense of superiority that we either are unaware of or can never admit to ourselves, we become highly fragile in conversations about race . . . Though white fragility is triggered by discomfort and anxiety, it is born of superiority and entitlement.[2]

White fragility—the anxiety with which white people approach situations where they might actually feel their race—keeps many white people from putting themselves in a position where they might be wrong so as to preserve their ego. Given that I don't commonly experience racial discomfort, it did give me anxiety to be in a situation where my ordinary sense of entitlement was muted. In this instance, my fear of being seen as an entitled white mother caused me to not sufficiently advocate for my son. While this may not be white fragility in a pure sense, if I find myself avoiding situations that require me to feel my race, I may be seduced into thinking that I am somehow inoculated from confronting race or building racial stamina.

Another blind spot for white people is their belief that as long as they take positions that have been characterized as liberal or progressive, they have this racism thing licked. In Chapter 2, we attempted to give you a snapshot of some of the history of race in the United States in a way that fosters real understanding of racism and how complicity with so-called race-neutral policies and practices today continues to perpetuate racist privilege and disadvantage. Misunderstanding and confusion about race and racism continue to divide the world. Even those who profess to be progressive-minded advocates of equity and inclusion may not recognize how their passivity or triumphalism perpetuates the negative impact of racist systems.

DiAngelo defines a white progressive as "any white person who thinks he or she is not racist or is less racist." That makes these "progressives" especially difficult for people of color to discuss race with because of the overpowering energy the self-proclaimed white progressives put into making sure that others see them as having achieved racial awareness.[3] As Shannon Sullivan explains in *Good White People: The Problem with Middle-Class White Anti-Racism*, many among the white middle-class consider themselves "the good whites" and separate themselves from less educated or working-class "bad whites" who they consider responsible for racial injustice.[4]

My husband, Mike, recently experienced this at, of all places, a summit on race. As close to two hundred people—a rich diversity of ethnicities, skin tones, religious beliefs, and neighborhoods— gathered for the explicit purpose of safe and organized dialogue, here comes Ms. White Woke Progressive with more words than work. She dominated the time and space, trying to prove how arrived and woke she was by telling everyone how frustrating it was for her to encounter and observe white privilege. She strove to demonstrate that because she could identify the imbalance of power in white spaces and openly point it out to the multiracial people seated around the table, she was one with them. As Mike recapped the evening to me, I felt myself cringing with discomfort. Mike was more than aggravated; he felt embarrassed and ashamed. We must resist the temptation to engage in behaviors and activities that merely create an image of progression, wokeness, or whatever the lexicon of the day but do nothing to further racial equity—and in fact perpetuate a racist agenda.

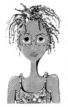 Often, white progressive organizers are quick to point out how their activism in their own self-inter-ests—be it feminist or class based—will benefit black people as well. This fails to recognize how black peo-ple's experience of class or gender is bound up in race and requires its own separate attention. But the harm done by this performance of allyship goes beyond neglect. For one thing, it under-mines the salience of the experiences of black people masking their realities. For another, it places an additional burden on people of color to continually set the record straight and educate others about their struggle for dignity and opportunity.

White privilege is so baked into American culture, and white Americans tend to be so invested in a narrative that justifies their privilege, that it's often difficult to recognize it as something that is wrong. I've heard it more times than I can count: "I know the system is flawed, but I didn't create it, and I want to believe that I wouldn't have." This narrative is reinforced by years of being told that black people who want to achieve do, and those who don't have squandered whatever opportunity is given to them. I have heard it in many forms. "Just look at how far *we've* come," as evi-denced by Barack Obama, Oprah Winfrey, and the slew of black doctors, lawyers, corporate executives, and entertainers, and in the frequently used "*They* have to pull themselves up by their boot-straps the way I did." White people will apply the inclusive lan-guage of *we* to the doers and connote the squanderers with a delin-eating *they* or *those people*. The achievements of some black people are used to justify the continuation of privilege for all white peo-ple, lulling us into a false belief that all is well. For others, they simply avoid the conversation of race altogether, which allows them to sidestep the necessity of confronting racist systems.

Progressives also are quick to remind me that they engage in a number of charitable activities that benefit black people, and black children in particular. While philanthropy certainly relieves the suffering of some, its goal is not necessarily racial equity for all. It may deflect attention from the fact that white people continue to reap the benefits of racist systems and soothes them into feeling less guilty about it. The haves can better enjoy the deliberate under-funding of predominantly black schools by supporting school fund-raisers to send black children back to dilapidated schools with new backpacks. An action to make an inequitable system more comfort-able for some helps those affected, but what does it do to build a better system? Recognizing privilege is a good start and dealing with the symptoms of racism by alleviating the suffering of a few can help, but addressing the cause and working to dismantle racist systems to achieve real racial equity is the endgame.

"People won't work to change a system that works for them," I heard a professor once proclaim, and my friends (both white and black) constantly remind me. "My kids' public school has a nice theater, two pools, a social worker on staff, computer tablets pro-vided to them by the school at no additional cost, and a library outfitted with new books and computers," they say. "I'm not giving up a tablet for my child so that the kid at the school five miles away with no library, no nurse, no books, and a building in disrepair can have a pencil." This is their position even if they don't express it in so many words, and even if they understand that racist policies created the inequity. Many readers of this book are in a unique position because sometimes their children will get the benefits of inheriting white privilege, while other times those same systems will deny them the advantages of their parents. Parents may feel like they are playing a lottery. But they are in a position to see more and advocate effectively for taking the uncertainty out of that lottery and securing a fairer world for their children.

How to Be an Antiracist by Ibram X. Kendi is a must-read. Kendi, one of the brilliant minds and prolific voices of this age, explains: "I had been taught that racist ideas cause racist policies. That igno-rance and hate cause racist ideas. That the root problem of racism is ignorance and hate. But that gets the chain of events exactly wrong. The root problem—from Prince Henry to President Trump—has always been the self-interest of racist power. Powerful economic, political, and cultural self-interest . . . Powerful and brilliant intellectuals . . . then produced racist ideas to justify the racist policies of their era, to redirect the blame for the era's racial inequities away from those policies and onto people."[5]

This is not just an American story. It's a human story. But in every story, there are people who work to dramatically change the social, political, and cultural system. For black people, this tradition reaches back to the ninth century and the Afro Iraqi Zanj Rebellion, and it includes Queen Nzinga resisting the Portuguese slave trade in Angola, Jamaica's Queen Nanny holding back the British, Toussaint L'Ouverture and the Haitian Revolution, and Nat Turner and resistance to enslavement in the United States. Other racial and ethnic groups have similar stories of oppression and triumph.

In crafting this book, we knew early on that it would challenge dualistic thinking and affirm evolutionary consciousness. The enthusiast, for example, can be shortsighted and the strong are often weak when it comes to calling out that which is wrong. However, many of us have been socialized to think dualistically; to believe if we accept anything about ourselves that hints of privilege or self-interest, that would be an admission that we are bad or racist, and so we deny it. Not one of us is all good or all bad and all of us are wonderful works in progress. Katie and I share a belief that people can evolve to embrace the age-old principle that life is not only about individual achievement, and we are only successful, we are only good, we are only righteous if our achievement contributes to the progress of the whole group. Everything we do, even if we do nothing, communicates either our affirmation or rejection of this principle. When we do nothing, it says that the existing system, even if cruel and unjust, is acceptable to us.

So what will you do? Will you commit to change and growth?

1. Will you support organizations that are working to change racist and oppressive systems, like those seeking to dismantle the current public education scheme and replace it with a fair funding formula?
2. Before you write a check or commit a vote, will you determine whether your local elected official is working to change racist policies or otherwise acting in the best interest of black people?
3. Will you refuse to lend financial support or patronage to efforts, whether film, television, or music, that perpetuate racist, stereotypical, imbalanced, or out-of-context images of black people or that make a mockery of those most affected by racist policies and actions?
4. If you live in a school district that is well resourced because of local wealth, would you be willing to give up some state funding to be redistributed to school districts with inadequate funding?
5. Will you do the hard work of agitating, influencing and persuading those who doubt that eradicating racism is just and right and in the best interest of all humanity?

The principles we have attempted to share in this book are as old as time and have been wrapped in the pleas of the abolitionist, the scholarship of the activist, the oratory of the theologian, and the words of novels, poems, "Letter from Birmingham Jail," and the Bible. This book is our effort to wrap these truths in our story, in our voice, and in our generation with the hope that you will view your place in the world with open eyes and then add your voice to the conversation. Gabriel is a gift that has illumined for us our place in the world and inspires us to experience a view we might not otherwise have known. When that happens, families, friendships, and villages have what it takes to straighten out each other's souls.

Notes

Chapter 1

1. Susan Smith et al., *Finding Families for African American Children: The Role of Race and Law in Adoption from Foster Care* (New York: Evan B. Donaldson Adoption Institute, 2008): 4, available at https://www.adoptioninstitute.org/publications/finding-families-for-african-american-children-the-role-of-race-law-in-adoption-from-foster-care.

2. Smith et al., *Finding Families for African American Children*, 12.

3. Ravinder Barn, "Doing the Right Thing: Transracial Adoption in the USA," *Ethnic and Racial Studies* 36, no. 8 (February 2013): 1273–1291.

4. Smith et al., *Finding Families for African American Children*, 12.

5. Rita J. Simon and Howard Altstein, *Transracial Adoptees and Their Families: A Study of Identity and Commitment* (New York: Praeger Publishers, 1987).

6. National Association of Black Social Workers (NABSW) Position Statement on Trans-Racial Adoptions, September 1972, accessed February 26, 2019, available at https://www.nabsw.org/page/PositionStatements.

7. Ibid.

8. Ibid.

9. Ibid.

10. Douglas R. Esten, "Transracial Adoption and the Multiethnic Placement Act of 1994," *Temple Law Review* 68 (Winter 1995): 1941–1997.

11. Ibid.

12. Lucille J. Grow and Deborah Shapiro, *Black Children—White Parents: A Study of Transracial Adoption* (New York: Child Welfare League of America, 1974); Dong Soo Kim, "How They Fared in American Homes: A Follow-Up Study of Adopted Korean Children," *Children Today* 6, no. 2 (March–April 1977): 2–6; Ruth G. McRoy et al., "Self-Esteem and Racial Identity in Transracial and Inracial Adoptees," *Social Work* 27, no. 6 (November 1982): 522–526; Ruth G. McRoy and Louis A. Zurcher, *Transracial and Inracial Adoptees: The Adolescent Years* (Springfield: Charles C. Thomas Publisher, 1983); William Feigelman and Arnold R. Silverman, *Chosen Children: New Patterns of Adoptive Relationships* (New York: Praeger, 1983); Joan F. Shireman and Penny R. Johnson, "A Longitudinal Study of Black Adoptions: Single Parent, Transracial, and Traditional," *Social Work* 31, no. 3 (May–June 1986): 172–176; Simon and Alstein, *Transracial Adoptees and Their Families*; Estela Andujo, "Ethnic Identity of Transethnically Adopted Hispanic Adolescents," *Social Work* 33, no. 6 (November–December 1988): 531–535; Marinus H. van IJzendoorn, "Adoptees Do Not Lack Self-Esteem: A Meta-Analysis of Studies on Self-Esteem of Transracial, International, and Domestic Adoptees," *Psychological Bulletin* 133, no. 6 (December 2007): 1067–1083; Gina Miranda Samuels, "'Being Raised by White People': Navigating Racial Difference Among Adopted Multiracial Adults," *Journal of Marriage and Family* 71 (February 2009): 80–94; M. Elizabeth Vonk, Jaegoo Lee, and Josie Crolley-Simic, "Cultural Socialization Practices in Domestic and International Transracial Adoption," *Adoption Quarterly* 13, no. 3 (July 2010): 222–247.

13. Smith et al., *Finding Families for African American Children*.

14. Leslie Doty Hollingsworth, "Effect of Transracial/Transethnic Adoption on Children's Racial and Ethnic Identity and Self-Esteem," *Marriage and Family Review* 25, no. 1–2 (September 1997): 99–130; Devon Brooks and Richard P. Barth, "Adult Transracial and Inracial Adoptees: Effects of Race, Gender, Adoptive Family Structure, and Placement History on Adjustment Outcomes," *American Journal of Orthopsychiatry* 69, no. 1 (January 1999): 87–99; van IJzendoorn, "Adoptees Do Not Lack Self-Esteem"; Samuels, "'Being Raised by White People'"; Vonk, Lee, and Crolley-Simic, "Cultural Socialization Practices"; Kathryn A. Sweeney, "How White Parents of Black and Multiracial Transracially Adopted Children Approach Racial Exposure and Neighborhood Choice," *Sociology of Race and Ethnicity* 3, no. 2 (April 2017): 236–252.

15. McRoy et al., "Self-Esteem and Racial Identity"; Andujo, "Ethnic Identity"; Amanda L. Baden, Lisa M. Treweeke, and Muninder K. Ahluwalia, "Reclaiming Culture: Reculturation of Transracial and Internation-

al Adoptees," *Journal of Counseling and Development* 90 (October 2012): 387–399; Emma R. Hamilton et al., "Identity Development in a Transracial Environment: Racial/Ethnic Minority Adoptees in Minnesota," *Adoption Quarterly* 18, no. 3 (February 2015): 217–233.

16. Smith et al., *Finding Families for African American Children*, 22.

17. Ibid.

18. Celia B. Fisher, Scyatta A. Wallace, and Rose E. Fenton, "Discrimination Distress during Adolescence," *Journal of Youth and Adolescence* 29, no. 6 (December 2000): 679–695.

19. Rita J. Simon and Rhonda M. Roorda, *In Their Parents' Voices: Reflections on Raising Transracial Adoptees* (New York: Columbia University Press, 2007).

20. NABSW, "Preserving African American Families," 1994, available at https://cdn.ymaws.com/www.nabsw.org/resource/collection/0D2D2404 -77EB-49B5-962E-7E6FADBF3D0D/Preserving_Families_of_African_ Ancestry.pdf. The more expansive 1994 document reinforced the 1972 position statement by stressing the following: (1) stopping unnecessary out-of-home placements, (2) reunification of children with parents, (3) placing children of African ancestry with relatives or unrelated families of the same race and culture for adoption, (4) addressing the barriers that prevent or discourage persons of African ancestry from adopting, (5) promoting culturally relevant agency practices, and (6) emphasizing that transracial adoption of an African-American child should only be considered after documented evidence of unsuccessful same race placements has been reviewed and supported by appropriate representatives of the African-American community (NABSW, 1994, p. 4).

21. Multiethnic Placement Act, 42 U.S.C. § 5115a (1994).

22. Chad Goller-Sojourner, "Transracial Family Coaching," accessed February 2, 2019, available at http://www.transracialfamilycoaching .com/.

23. NPR Staff, "Growing Up 'White,' Transracial Adoptee Learned to Be Black," *NPR*, January 26, 2014, available at https://www.npr.org/ 2014/01/26/266434175/growing-up-white-transracial-adoptee-learned -to-be-black.

24. Chad Goller-Sojourner, "Transracial Family Coaching."

25. John Raible, "About John," accessed February 2, 2019, available at https://johnraible.wordpress.com/about-john-w-raible/dr-raibles-writ ings.

26. Ibid.

27. Smith et al., *Finding Families for African American Children*.

Chapter 2

1. Barack Obama, *Dreams from My Father: A Story of Race and Inheritance* (New York: Three Rivers Press, 2004), 89.

2. Camara Phyllis Jones et al., "Using Socially Assigned Race to Probe White Advantages in Health Status," *Ethnicity and Disease* 18, no. 4 (Autumn 2008): 496–504.

3. Molefi Kete Asante, "Contours of the African American Culture," 2009, accessed February 23, 2019, available at http://www.asante.net/articles/12/contours-of-the-african-american-culture.

4. A. Leon Higginbotham Jr., *In the Matter of Color: Race and the American Legal Process: The Colonial Period* (Oxford: Oxford University Press, 1978), 20.

5. John Hope Franklin, in United States Commission on Civil Rights, *Freedom to the Free* (Washington, D.C.: U.S. Government Printing Office, 1963), 71.

6. Higginbotham, *In the Matter of Color*, 39.

7. June Purcell Guild, *Black Laws of Virginia: A Summary of the Legislative Acts of Virginia Concerning Negroes from Earliest Times to the Present* (New York: Negro University Press, 1969), 45.

8. Audrey Smedley and Brian D. Smedley, "Race as Biology Is Fiction, Racism as a Social Problem Is Real," *American Psychologist* 60, no. 1 (January 2005): 19.

9. James Baldwin, *If Beale Street Could Talk* (New York: The Dial Press, 1974).

10. U.S. Constitution, art. I, § 2, cl. 3.

11. U.S. Constitution, art. IV, § 2, cl. 3.

12. U.S. Constitution, art. I, § 9, cl. 1.

13. The 1776 Pennsylvania Constitution provided:

> A school or schools shall be established in each county by the legislature, for the convenient instruction of youth, with such salaries to the masters paid by the public, as may enable them to instruct youth at low prices.

The state constitution of 1790 contained a similar provision:

> The legislature shall, as soon as conveniently may be, provide, by law, for the establishment of schools throughout the state, in such manner that the poor may be taught gratis.

14. An Act for the Gradual Abolition of Slavery (1780).

15. Laws of Pennsylvania, § 24 (1854).

16. *Debates of the Convention to Amend the Constitution of Pennsylvania*, Volume 2 (Harrisburg: Benjamin Singerly, 1873), 426.

17. Laws of Pennsylvania, P.L. 76 (June 8, 1881).

18. U.S. Department of Education, "The Federal Role in Education," accessed July 31, 2019, available at http://www2.ed.gov/about/overview/fed/role.html.

19. For more information about the history of education funding in Pennsylvania, check out Education Law Center, "Money Matters in Education Justice: Addressing Racial and Class Inequities in Pennsylvania's School Funding System," March 2017, available at https://www.elc-pa.org/wp-content/uploads/2017/03/Education-Justice-Report.pdf.

20. Dred Scott v. Sandford, 60 U.S. 393 (1857).

21. Dred Scott, 60 U.S. 393, 407.

22. Ibid.

23. Declaration of Independence (1776).

24. Dred Scott, 60 U.S. 393, 410.

25. Emancipation Proclamation (1863).

26. U.S. Constitution, amend. XIII.

27. U.S. Constitution, amend. XIV.

28. To learn more about the Reconstruction era, check out Maulana Karenga, *Introduction to Black Studies* (Los Angeles: University of Sankore Press, 2002), 165; "Eyes on the Prize," American Experience, accessed July 31, 2019, available at https://www.pbs.org/wgbh/americanexperience/films/eyesontheprize.

29. Karenga, *Introduction to Black Studies*, 165.

30. Plessy v. Ferguson, 163 U.S. 537 (1896).

31. Plessy, 163 U.S. 537, 551.

32. Karenga, *Introduction to Black Studies*, 165–167.

33. For facts and general information about the Great Depression, visit https://www.history.com/topics/great-depression/great-depression-history.

34. Ira Katznelson, *When Affirmative Action Was White: An Untold History of Racial Inequality in Twentieth-Century America* (New York: W. W. Norton, 2005).

35. Katznelson, *When Affirmative Action Was White*, 23.

36. To review risk assessment maps for more than one hundred communities, visit https://www.policymap.com.

37. To learn more about the impact of racially discriminatory federal housing policies, check out Ta-Nehisi Coates, "The Case for Reparations," *The Atlantic*, June 2014, available at http://www.theatlantic.com/maga zine/archive/2014/06/the-case-for-reparations/361631.

38. David McAllister, "Realtors and Racism in Working-Class Philadelphia, 1945–1970," in *African American Urban History since World War II*, eds. Kenneth L. Kusmer and Joe W. Trotter (Chicago: University of Chicago Press, 2009), 123–141.

39. Andrew Wiese, "'The House I Live In': Race, Class, and African American Suburban Dreams in the Postwar United States," in *African American Urban History*, 160–178.

40. McAllister, "Realtors and Racism," 123–141. Also check out: "Historian Says Don't 'Sanitize' How Our Government Created Ghettos," *NPR*, May 14, 2015, available at https://www.npr.org/2015/05/14/406699264/historian-says-dont-sanitize-how-our-government-created-the-ghettos.

41. Chuck Collins et al., "Dreams Deferred: How Enriching the 1% Widens the Racial Wealth Divide," Institute for Policy Studies, January 15, 2019, 13, available at https://ips-dc.org/wp-content/uploads/2019/01/IPS_RWD-Report_FINAL-1.15.19.pdf.

42. Ibid., 9.

43. Ibid.

44. Brown v. Board of Education I, 387 U.S. 483 (1954).

45. Plessy, 163 U.S. 537 (1896).

46. Brown v. Board of Education II, 349 U.S. 294 (1955).

47. Charles Ogletree Jr., *All Deliberate Speed: Reflections on the First Half Century of Brown v. Board of Education* (New York: W. W. Norton, 2004), 259.

48. Ogletree, *All Deliberate Speed*, 260.

49. Gary Orfield, John Kucsera, and Genevieve Siegel-Hawley, "E Pluribus . . . Separation: Deepening Double Segregation for More Students," The Civil Rights Project, September 19, 2012, 10, available at http://civ ilrightsproject.ucla.edu/research/k-12-education/integration-and-di versity/mlk-national/e-pluribus...separation-deepening-double-segrega tion-for-more-students.

50. Executive Order 10925 (1961).

51. Charles Whalen and Barbara Whalen, *The Longest Debate: A Legislative History of the 1964 Civil Rights Act* (New York: New American Library, 1985).

52. Whalen and Whalen, *The Longest Debate*, xviii.

53. Whalen and Whalen, *The Longest Debate*, 21.

54. Civil Rights Act of 1964, Title VII, 42 U.S.C. § 2000e et seq.

55. Whalen and Whalen, *The Longest Debate*, x.

56. Bureau of Labor Statistics, "Labor Force Characteristics by Race and Ethnicity, 2017," August 2018, Table 8, available at https://www.bls.gov/opub/reports/race-and-ethnicity/2017/home.htm.

57. Ibid., Table 8.

58. Ibid., Table 17.

59. Collins et al., "Dreams Deferred," 13.

60. Regents of the University of California v. Bakke, 438 U.S. 265 (1978).

61. Gratz v. Bollinger, 539 U.S. 244 (2003).

62. Grutter v. Bollinger, 539 U.S. 306 (2003).

63. Fisher v. University of Texas at Austin I, 570 U.S. ___, 133 S. Ct. 2411 (2013); Fisher v. University of Texas at Austin II, 579 U.S. ___(2016).

64. Fisher II, 579 U.S. at ___(slip op., at 7).

65. Bureau of Labor Statistics, "Labor Force Characteristics," Table 6.

66. Ibid., Table 17.

67. "School Spending," Commonwealth Foundation, accessed July 31, 2019, available at http://www.openpagov.org/education_revenue_and_expenses.asp. These 2015–2016 figures reflect a troubling trend of substantially lower investment in education for students at predominantly black schools in relation to their white counterparts. To learn more about education funding in Pennsylvania, visit the Education Law Center (https://www.elc-pa.org) and the Public Interest Law Center (https://www.pubintlaw.org).

68. Anthony P. Carnevale and Jeff Strohl, *Separate and Unequal: How Higher Education Reinforces the Intergenerational Reproduction of White Racial Privilege* (Washington, D.C.: Georgetown Public Policy Institute Center on Education and the Workforce, 2013), 7.

69. Carnevale and Strohl, *Separate and Unequal*, 7.

Chapter 3

1. Karen T. Craddock, "'It's Not in Our Head' . . . and yet Pain Is in Our Brain: Why Racialized Exclusion Hurts and How We Can Remain Resilient," blog post, January 19, 2019, accessed February 3, 2019, available at https://www.embracerace.org/blog/its-not-in-our-head-and-yet-pain-is-in-our-brain-why-racialized-exclusion-hurts-and-how-we-can-remain

-resilient; N. I. Eisenberger and M. D. Lieberman, "Why Rejection Hurts: A Common Neural Alarm System for Physical and Social Pain," *TRENDS in Cognitive Sciences* 8, no. 7 (2004): 294–300.

2. Craddock, "It's Not in Our Head."

3. Kate M. Wegmann, "'His Skin Doesn't Match What He Wants to Do': Children's Perceptions of Stereotype Threat," *American Journal of Orthopsychiatry* 87, no. 6 (2017): 615–625.

4. William E. Cross, *Shades of Back: Diversity in African-American Identity* (Philadelphia: Temple University Press, 1991); Madonna G. Constantine et al., "An Overview of Black Racial Identity Theories: Limitations and Considerations for Future Theoretical Conceptualizations," *Applied and Preventive Psychology* 7, no. 2 (1998): 95–99.

5. Manning Marable, *Black Liberation in Conservative America* (Boston: South End, 1997), 195.

6. Keyiona Ritchey, "Black Identity Development," *The Vermont Connection* 35 (2014): 100; Ronald Sentwali Bakari, "African American Racial Identity Development in Predominantly White Institutions: Challenges for Student Development Professionals," *Different Perspectives on Majority Rules* (April 1997): 1.

7. Cyndy R. Snyder, "Racial Socialization in Cross-Racial Families," *Journal of Black Psychology* 38, no. 2 (2012): 228–253.

8. Molefi Kete Asante, *The History of Africa: The Quest for Eternal Harmony* (New York: Routledge, 2019), xii.

9. Ibid., xii.

10. Georg Hegel, *The Philosophy of History* (New York: Cosimo, 2007), 99.

11. Ibid., 99.

12. Ibid., 98.

13. Ibid., 99.

14. Ibram X. Kendi, *Stamped from the Beginning: The Definitive History of Racist Ideas in America* (New York: Nation Books, 2016).

15. The Opportunity Agenda, "Media Representations and Impact on the Lives of Black Men and Boys," October 2011, 24, available at http://racialequitytools.org/resourcefiles/Media-Impact-onLives-of-Black-Men-and-Boys-OppAgenda.pdf; Rosalee A. Clawson and Rakuya Trice, "Poverty as We Know It: Media Portrayals of the Poor," *Public Opinion Quarterly* 64, no. 1 (March 2000): 53, 56–67; Rosalee A. Clawson, Mark Franciose, and Adam Scheidt, "The Racialized Portrayal of Poverty," presentation, Annual Meeting of the Midwest Political Science Association, Chicago, IL, April 12, 2007.

16. Robert M. Entman and Kimberly A. Gross, "Race to Judgement: Stereotyping Media and Criminal Defendants," *Law and Contemporary Problems* 71, no. 4 (Fall 2008): 98; Travis L. Dixon and Daniel Linz, "Race and the Misrepresentation of Victimization on Local Television News," *Communication Research* 27, no. 5 (October 2000): 559–560.

17. "Portrayal and Perception: Two Audits of News Media Reporting on African American Men and Boys," Heinz Endowments' African American Men and Boys Task Force, November 2011, available at www.heinz.org/ UserFiles/Library/AAMB-MediaReport.pdf.

18. U.S. Census Bureau, Current Population Survey, 1968 through 2017, Annual Social and Economic Supplements.

19. "By the Numbers: More Black Men in Prison Than in College? Think Again," American Council on Education, available at Fall 2012, https:// www.acenet.edu/the-presidency/columns-and-features/Pages/By-the -Numbers-More-Black-Men-in-Prison-Than-in-College-Think-Again -.aspx; U.S. Department of Justice, Bureau of Justice Statistics Publications, National Prisoner Statistics Program, 1978–2013; U.S. Department of Education, Institute of Education Sciences, National Center for Education Statistics, Table 306.10, 2018, available at https://nces.ed.gov/programs/ digest/d18/ta bles/dt18_306.10.asp.

20. Anthony G. Greenwald, Mark A. Oakes, and Hunter G. Hoffman, "Targets of Discrimination: Effects of Race on Responses to Weapons Holders," *Journal of Experimental Social Psychology* 39, no. 4 (July 2003): 399–405.

21. Nielsen, "State of the Media Trends in TV Viewing—2011 TV Upfronts," April 2011, available at https://www.nielsen.com/wp-content/ uploads/sites/3/2019/04/State-of-the-Media-2011-TV-Upfronts.pdf.

22. The Opportunity Agenda, "Media Representations and Impact," 29–30; Alexis S. Tan and Gerdean Tan, "Television Use and Self-Esteem of Blacks," *Journal of Communication* 29, no. 1 (March 1979): 129–135.

23. Vittorio Gallese, as quoted in Lea Winerman, "The Mind's Mirror," *Monitor* 36, no. 9 (October 2005): 48, available at https://www.apa.org/ monitor/oct05/mirror.aspx.

24. Steven J. Spencer, Christine Logel, and Paul G. Davies, "Stereotype Threat," *Annual Review of Psychology* 67 (2016): 422.

25. Karen Valby, "The Realities of Raising a Kid of a Different Race," *Time Magazine*, February 1, 2015, available at http://time.com/the-reali ties-of-raising-a-kid-of-a-different-race.

26. Eddie Moore Jr., Ali Michael, and Marguerite Penick-Parks, eds., *The Guide for White Women Who Teach Black Boys* (Thousand Oaks: Corwin, 2018).

27. Molefi Kete Asante, *Afrocentricity: The Theory of Social Change* (Chicago: African American Images, 2003): 2.

28. Joseph E. Flynn Jr., "White Fatigue: Naming the Challenge in Moving from an Individual to a Systemic Understanding of Racism," *Multicultural Perspectives* 17, no. 3 (August 2015): 120.

29. Phillip J. Bowman and Cleopatra Howard, "Race-Related Socialization, Motivation, and Academic Achievement: A Study of Black Youths in Three-Generation Families," *Journal of the American Academy of Child and Adolescent Psychiatry* 24, no. 2 (March 1985): 134–141; Ardis C. Martin, "Television Media as a Potential Negative Factor in the Racial Identity Development of African American Youth," *Academic Psychiatry* 32, no. 4 (July 2008): 338–342; Colleen Butler-Sweet, "'A Healthy Black Identity' Transracial Adoption, Middle-Class Families, and Racial Socialization," *Journal of Comparative Family Studies* 42, no. 2 (January–February 2011): 193–198; Ashley B. Evans et al., "Racial Socialization as a Mechanism for Positive Development Among African American Youth," *Child Development Perspective* 6, no. 3 (February 2012): 251–257.

30. Cheikh Anta Diop, *Civilization or Barbarism: An Authentic Anthropology* (Brooklyn: Lawrence Hill Books, 1991), 2–3.

31. Asante, *The History of Africa*, Appendix 1.

32. Asante, *Afrocentricity*, 65.

33. Wikipedia, "List of Museums Focused on African Americans," accessed June 17, 2019, available at https://en.wikipedia.org/wiki/List_of_museums_focused_on_African_Americans.

34. Kwame Gyekye, *An Essay on African Philosophical Thought: The Akan Conceptual Scheme* (Philadelphia: Temple University Press, 1987), 191.

35. Ibid., 191.

36. The Official Kwanzaa Website, "Kwanzaa," accessed June 17, 2019, available at http://www.officialkwanzaawebsite.org/index.shtml.

37. The African American Literature Book Club, accessed October 14, 2019, available at https://aalbc.com/books/children.php.

38. Gyekye, *An Essay on African Philosophical Thought*, 189.

39. Styles 4 Kidz, NFP is a 501(c)(3) nonprofit organization that provides high-quality, compassionate hair care education and services for African American kids in foster care and transracial adoptive families. For more information, check out https://www.styles4kidz.org/programs.

40. Richard Lischer, "The Music of Martin Luther King, Jr.," in *This Is How We Flow: Rhythm in Black Cultures*, ed. Angela M.S. Nelson (Columbia: University of South Carolina Press, 1999), 59.

41. Valby, "The Realities."

Chapter 4

1. Kathy Hardie-Williams, "The Importance of Community Support in Raising Children," *Good Therapy*, May 3, 2016, accessed November 1, 2019, available at https://www.goodtherapy.org/blog/importance-of-community -support-in-raising-children-0503165; Frederic Laloux, "We Are Wired to Raise Children in Community," *Medium*, December 11, 2017, accessed November 1, 2019, available at https://medium.com/@fredlaloux/we-are -wired-to-raise-children-in-community-103cd4e9e9bf.

2. J. Eric Oliver and Tali Mendelberg, "Reconsidering the Environmental Determinants of White Racial Attitudes," *American Journal of Political Science* 44, no. 3 (July 2000): 574–589

3. Michelle Obama, *Becoming* (New York: Crown Publishing, 2018): 3.

Chapter 5

1. Eddie Glaude Jr. quote from an interview on *The Ezra Klein Show,* "How Whiteness Distorts Our Democracy (and the Ideas That Animate Our Democracy)," accessed April 4, 2019, available at https://www.stitch er.com/podcast/vox/the-ezra-klein-show/e/59837986.

2. Brian D. Smedley, Adrienne Y. Stith, and Alan R. Nelson, eds., *Unequal Treatment: Confronting Racial and Ethnic Disparities in Health Care* (Washington, D.C.: Institute of Medicine [US] Committee on Understanding and Eliminating Racial and Ethnic Disparities in Health Care, National Academies Press, 2013).

3. Louise Wang et al., "Health Outcomes in US Children with Abdominal Pain at Major Emergency Departments Associated with Race and Socioeconomic Status," *PLoS ONE* 10, no. 8 (August 2015): 1–17; Chet D. Schrader and Lawrence M. Lewis, "Racial Disparity in Emergency Department Triage," *Journal of Emergency Medicine* 44, no. 2 (2013): 511–518; Nancy Sonnenfeld et al., "Emergency Department Volume and Racial and Ethnic Differences in Waiting Times in the United States," *Medical Care* 50 (April 2002): 335–341; Paula A. Johnson et al., "Effect of Race on the Presentation and Management of Patients with Acute Chest Pain," *Annals of Internal Medicine* 118, no. 8 (April 1993): 593–601.

4. Smedley et al., "Unequal Treatment: Confronting Racial and Ethnic Disparities in Health Care."

5. Wang et al., "Health Outcomes in US Children with Abdominal Pain at Major Emergency Departments Associated with Race and Socioeconomic Status."

6. Ibid.

7. Allana Akhtar, "New York Is Investigating UnitedHealth's Use of a Medical Algorithm That Steered Black Patients Away from Getting Higher-Quality Care," *Business Insider,* October 28, 2019, available at https://www.businessinsider.com/an-algorithm-treatment-to-white-patients-over-sicker-black-ones-2019-10.

8. Ziad Obermeyer et al., "Dissecting Racial Bias in an Algorithm Used to Manage the Health of Populations," *Science* 366 (October 2019): 447.

9. NPR Staff, "Growing Up 'White,' Transracial Adoptee Learned to Be Black," *NPR,* January 26, 2014, available at https://www.npr.org/2014/01/26/266434175/growing-up-white-transracial-adoptee-learned-to-be-black.

10. Teletia R. Taylor et al., "Racial Discrimination and Breast Cancer Incidence in US Black Women: The Black Women's Health Study," *American Journal of Epidemiology* 166, no. 1 (July 2007): 46–54.

11. Maria Trent, Danielle G. Dooley, and Jacqueline Dougé, "The Impact of Racism on Child and Adolescent Health," *Pediatrics* 144, no. 2 (August 2019).

12. Wegmann, "His Skin Doesn't Match What He Wants to Do."

13. Priscilla Dass-Brailsford, *A Practical Approach to Trauma: Empowering Interventions* (Thousand Oaks: Sage Publications, 2007).

14. Ibid.

15. Trent et al., "The Impact of Racism on Child and Adolescent Health."

Chapter 6

1. Ary Spatig-Amerikaner, "Unequal Education—Federal Loophole Enables Lower Spending on Students of Color," Center for American Progress, August 2012, accessed on November 1, 2019, available at https://www.americanprogress.org/wp-content/uploads/2012/08/UnequalEducation.pdf.

2. Dale Mezzacappa, "Democratic Legislators Say Fixing School Funding Is a Moral Imperative," *The Notebook,* January 25, 2019, accessed June 25, 2019, available at https://whyy.org/articles/democratic-legislators-say-fixing-school-funding-is-a-moral-imperative._

3. Research for Action is a Philadelphia-based nonprofit education research organization. It was founded in 1992 by Drs. Eva Gold and Jolley Bruce Christman with a commitment to conducting education research that explored the complexities of education reform initiatives in Philadelphia and provided education stakeholders with common-sense research to inform their initiatives. For more information, check out https://www.researchforaction.org.

4. https://www.researchforaction.org/publications/unequal-access-to-ed ucational-opportunity-among-pennsylvanias-high-school-students/.

5. Moore Jr., Michael, and Penick-Parks, eds., *The Guide for White Women Who Teach Black Boys*.

6. https://alimichael.org/anti-racism-resources-for-teachers.

7. "The State of Racial Diversity in the Educator Workforce," U.S. Department of Education, Office of Planning, Evaluation and Policy Development, Policy and Program Studies Service, 2016, accessed June 25, 2019, available at http://www2.ed.gov/rschstat/eval/highered/racial-diversity/ state-racial-diversityworkforce.pdf.

8. Ibid.

9. Seth Gershenson et al., "The Long-Run Impacts of Same-Race Teachers," National Bureau of Economic Research, November 2018, accessed June 25, 2019, available at https://www.nber.org/papers/w25254.pdf.

10. U.S. Department of Education, "The State of Racial Diversity in the Educator Workforce."

11. "The Condition of College and Career Readiness—African American Students 2015," Report from ACT and the United Negro College Fund, 2015, accessed June 25, 2019, available at https://www.uncf.org/wp-con tent/uploads/PDFs/6201-CCCR-African-American-2015.pdf.

12. Seth Gershenson, Stephen B. Holt, and Nicholas W. Papageorge, "Who Believes in Me? The Effect of Student-Teacher Demographic Match on Teacher Expectations," *Economics of Education Review* 52 (June 2016): 222.

13. Anna Egalite, Brian Kisida, and Marcus A. Winters, "Representation in the Classroom: The Effect of Own-Race Teachers on Student Achievement," *Economics of Education Review* 45 (April 2015); Gershenson et al., "Who Believes in Me?"; Gershenson et al., "The Long-Run Impacts of Same-Race Teachers."

14. Jill Rosen, "Black Students Who Have One Black Teacher Are More Likely to Go to College," November 12, 2018, accessed November 1, 2019, available at https://hub.jhu.edu/2018/11/12/black-students-black-teach ers-college-gap.

15. "Civil Rights Data Collection, Data Snapshot: School Discipline," U.S. Department of Education Office for Civil Rights, Issue Brief No. 1, March 2014, accessed June 23, 2019, available at https://ocrdata.ed.gov/ downloads/crdc-school-discipline-snapshot.pdf.

16. "Civil Rights Data Collection, Data Snapshot: School Discipline," U.S. Department of Education Office for Civil Rights.

17. Ibid.

18. "Let Her Learn: Stopping School Pushout," National Women's Law Center, National Clearinghouse on Supporting School Discipline, published 2017, August 28, 2019, available at https://supportiveschooldiscipline.org/learn/reference-guides/pushout.

19. "Black Girls Matter: Pushed Out, Overpoliced and Underprotected," African American Policy Forum and Center for Intersectionality and Social Policy Studies, 2015, accessed June 23, 2019, available at http://static1.squarespace.com/static/53f20d90e4b0b80451158d8c/t/54d2d22ae4b00c506cffe978/1423102506084/BlackGirlsMatter_Report.pdf.

20. Anne Gregory and Edward Fergus, "Social and Emotional Learning and Equity in School Discipline," *Future of Children* 27, no. 1 (January 2017): 122.

21. Moore Jr., Michael, and Penick-Parks, eds., *The Guide for White Women Who Teach Black Boys.*

22. Ibid., 95.

23. Steven J. Spencer, Christine Logel, and Paul G. Davies, "Stereotype Threat," *The Annual Review of Psychology*, 67 (2016): 420–421.

24. Wegmann, "His Skin Doesn't Match What He Wants to Do."

25. Spencer et al., "Stereotype Threat," 418.

26. Ibid.

27. The Higher Education Act of 1965, as amended.

28. National Center for Education Statistics, "Fast Facts: Historically Black Colleges and Universities," July 3, 2019, available at https://nces.ed.gov/fastfacts/display.asp?id=667. National Center for Education Statistics (NCES) is the primary federal entity for collecting and analyzing data related to education in the United States and other nations. NCES is located within the U.S. Department of Education and the Institute of Education Sciences. NCES fulfills a congressional mandate to collect, collate, analyze, and report complete statistics on the condition of American education; conduct and publish reports; and review and report on education activities internationally.

29. David Wall Rice and Shaun R. Harper, "Stop Asking if HBCUs Are Relevant," *Ebony Magazine*, August 26, 2019, available at https://www.ebony.com/news/stop-asking-if-hbcus-are-relevant-392.

30. United Negro College Fund, "The Impact of HBCUs on Diversity in Stem Fields," February 4, 2019, accessed July 3, 2019, available at https://www.uncf.org/the-latest/the-impact-of-hbcus-on-diversity-in-stem-fields.

31. United Negro College Fund, "The Impact of HBCUs on Diversity in Stem Fields."

32. "Civil Rights Data Collection, Data Snapshot: School Discipline," U.S. Department of Education Office for Civil Rights.

Chapter 7

1. Karen Valby, "The Realities of Raising a Kid of a Different Race," *Time Magazine*, February 1, 2015, available at http://time.com/the-realities-of-raising-a-kid-of-a-different-race.

2. Muhammad Ahmad, *We Will Return in the Whirlwind: Black Radical Organizations 1960–1975* (Chicago: Charles H. Kerr Publishing, 2008): 171.

3. Ibid., 172.

4. Ibid., 186.

5. Ward Churchill and Jim Vander Wall, *Agents of Repression: The FBI's Secret Wars Against the Black Panther Party and the American Indian Movement* (Boston: South End Press, 1988): 77.

6. Frank Donner, *Protectors of Privilege: Red Squads and Police Repression in Urban America* (Berkeley: University of California, 1990): 180.

7. Chris Booker, "Lumpenization: A Critical Error of the Black Panther Party," in *The Black Panther Party Reconsidered*, ed. Charles Jones (Baltimore: Black Classic Press, 1998): 356.

8. Omari L. Dyson, "The Life and Work of the Philadelphia Black Panthers: The Curricular and Pedagogical Implications of Their Social Transformation Efforts" (Ph.D. diss., Purdue University, 2008): 137.

9. Ibid., 142.

10. Ibid., 146.

11. Omari L. Dyson, Kevin L. Brooks, and Judson L. Jeffries, "Brotherly Love Can Kill You: The Philadelphia Branch of the Black Panther Party," in *Comrades: A Local History of the Black Panther Party*, ed. Judson L. Jeffries (Bloomington: Indiana University Press, 2007): 218.

12. Ibid., 219.

13. Ibid., 214–215.

14. United Press International, "Panthers' Survivors Win Suit," *Philadelphia Inquirer*, March 1, 1983.

15. Rory Kramer and Brianna Remster, "Stop, Frisk, and Assault? Racial Disparities in Police Use of Force During Investigatory Stops," *Law and Society Review* 52, no. 4 (2018): 960.

16. Ibid.

17. Ibid.

18. Sheri Levy, Steven Stroessner, and Carol Dweck, "Stereotype Formation and Endorsement: The Role of Implicit Theories," *Journal of Personality and Social Psychology* 74, no. 6 (1998): 1421–1436; Phillip Atiba Goff et al., "The Essence of Innocence: Consequences of Dehumanizing Black Children," *Journal of Personality and Social Psychology* 106, no. 4 (2014): 529.

19. Phillip Atiba Goff et al., "The Essence of Innocence," 526–545.

20. Ibid., 527.

21. Priscilla Gibson et al., "A Mixed Methods Study of Black Girls' Vulnerability to Out-of-School Suspensions: The Intersection of Race and Gender," *Children and Youth Services Review* 102 (2019): 169–176.

22. James C. Barnes and Ryan T. Motz, "Reducing Racial Inequalities in Adulthood Arrest by Reducing Inequalities in School Discipline: Evidence from the School-to-Prison Pipeline," *Developmental Psychology* 54, no. 12 (2018): 2329–2330.

23. Harry Wilson, "Turning off the School-to-Prison Pipeline," *Reclaiming Children and Youth* 23, no. 1 (Spring 2014): 49–53.

24. Executive Order 13684: Establishment of the President's Task Force on 21st Century Policing, December 2014, accessed September 2019, available at https://www.hsdl.org/?abstract&did=760795.

25. Ibid.

26. President's Task Force on 21st Century Policing, *Final Report of the President's Task Force on 21st Century Policing*, May 2015, accessed November 1, 2019, available at https://cops.usdoj.gov/ric/Publications/cops-p311-pub.pdf.

27. Barnes and Motz, "Reducing Racial Inequalities in Adulthood Arrest by Reducing Inequalities in School Discipline," 2336.

28. "Dear Child—When Black Parents Have to Give 'The Talk,'" accessed June 2019, available at https://www.youtube.com/watch?v=Mkw 1CetjWwI; Clint Smith, "How to Raise a Black Son in America," TED2015, accessed June 2019, available at https://www.ted.com/talks/clint_smith_how_to_raise_a_black_son_in_america/discussion; "Black Americans Turn to Their Children to Give 'The Talk,'" *ABC News*, accessed June 2019, available at https://www.youtube.com/watch?v=HX8zamQ5Yxw; "Black Parents Describe 'The Talk' They Give to Their Children about Police," *New York Times*, August 2016, accessed June 2019, available at https://www.vox.com/2016/8/8/12401792/police-black-parents-the-talk; Natalie Hopkinson, "I Refuse to Give My Black Son 'The Talk,'" *Huffington Post*, September 9, 2018, accessed November 1, 2019, available at https://www.huffingtonpost.com/entry/opinion-kaepernick-police-brutality-driving-black-men_us_5b9185c2e4b0cf7b003df96f; Issac Bailey, "I Refuse to

Have 'The Talk' with My Black Son," *Politico*, December 1, 2015, accessed November 1, 2019, available at https://www.politico.com/magazine/sto ry/2015/12/why-i-refuse-to-have-the-talk-with-my-black-son-213406.

29. Tamir Rice Safety Handbook, ACLU Ohio, accessed December 2019, available at https://www.acluohio.org/tamirricesafetyhandbook.

30. Maralee Bradley, "Dear White Parents of My Black Child's Friends: I Need Your Help," ScaryMommy.com, accessed November 1, 2019, avail able at https://www.scarymommy.com/black-child-friends.

Chapter 8

1. Beverly Daniel Tatum, *Why Are All the Black Kids Sitting Together in the Cafeteria? And Other Conversations about Race* (New York: Basic Books, 2017).

2. Robin DiAngelo, *White Fragility: Why It's So Hard for White People to Talk about Racism* (Boston: Beacon Press, 2018): 1–2.

3. DiAngelo, *White Fragility*, 5.

4. Shannon Sullivan, *Good White People: The Problem with Middle-Class White Anti-Racism* (Albany: SUNY Press, 2014).

5. Ibram X. Kendi, *How to Be an Antiracist* (New York: One Book, 2019): 42–43.

Further Reading

ACLU Ohio. 2019. "Tamir Rice Safety Handbook." Accessed December 2019. Available at www.acluohio.org/tamirricesafetyhandbook.

African American Policy Forum and Center for Intersectionality and Social Policy Studies. 2015. *Black Girls Matter: Pushed Out, Overpoliced and Underprotected*. Accessed June 23, 2019. Available at http://static1.square space.com/static/53f20d90e4b0b80451158d8c/t/54d2d22ae4b00c 506cffe978/1423102506084/BlackGirlsMatter_Report.pdf.

Alexander, Michelle. 2012. *The New Jim Crow: Mass Incarceration in the Age of Colorblindness*. New York: The New Press.

Asante, Molefi Kete. 2003. *Afrocentricity: The Theory of Social Change*. Chicago: African American Images.

———. 2012. *The African American People: A Global History*. New York: Routledge.

———. 2019. *The History of Africa: The Quest for Eternal Harmony*. New York: Routledge.

Bailey, Issac. 2015. "I Refuse to Have 'The Talk' with My Black Son." Politico, December 1. Accessed November 1, 2019. Available at https://www .politico.com/magazine/story/2015/12/why-i-refuse-to-have-the -talk-with-my-black-son-213406.

Baldwin, James. 1974. *If Beale Street Could Talk*. New York: The Dial Press.

Barnes, James C., and Ryan T. Motz. 2018. "Reducing Racial Inequalities in Adulthood Arrest by Reducing Inequalities in School Discipline: Evidence from the School-to-Prison Pipeline." *Developmental Psychology* 54 (12): 2328–2340.

Bradley, Maralee. n.d. ScaryMommy.com. Accessed November 1, 2019. Available at https://www.scarymommy.com/black-child-friends.

Carnevale, Anthony P., and Jeff Strohl. 2013. *Separate and Unequal: How Higher Education Reinforces the Intergenerational Reproduction of White Racial Privilege.* Washington, D.C.: Georgetown Public Policy Institute Center on Education and the Workforce.

Coates, Ta-Nehisi. 2014. "The Case for Reparations." *The Atlantic.* June. Available at http://www.theatlantic.com/magazine/archive/2014/06/the-case-for-reparations/361631.

Cross, William E. 1991. *Shades of Black: Diversity in African-American Identity.* Philadelphia: Temple Press.

DiAngelo, Robin. 2018. *White Fragility: Why It's So Hard for White People to Talk about Racism.* Boston: Beacon Press.

Dovidio, John F. 2001. "On the Nature of Contemporary Prejudice: The Third Wave." *Journal of Social Issues* (57) 4: 829–849.

Egalite, Anna, Brian Kisida, and Marcus A. Winters. 2015. "Representation in the Classroom: The Effect of Own-Race Teachers on Student Achievement." *Economics of Education Review* 45–52 (June).

Epp, Charles R., Steven Maynard-Moody, and Donald Haider-Harkel. 2014. *Pulled Over: How Police Stops Define Race and Citizenship.* Chicago: University of Chicago.

Forman, James, Jr. 2017. *Locking Up Our Own: Crime and Punishment in Black America.* New York: Farrar, Straus, and Giroux.

Gershenson, Seth, Cassandra M. D. Hart, Joshua Hyman, Constance Lindsay, and Nicholas W. Papageorge. 2018. "The Long-Run Impacts of Same-Race Teachers." *National Bureau of Economic Research Working Paper Series.* Cambridge, MA, November. Accessed June 2019. Available at https://www.nber.org/papers/w25254.pdf.

Gibson, Priscilla, Wendy Haight, Minhae Cho, Ndilimeke J.C. Nashandi, and Young Ji Yoon. 2019. "A Mixed Methods Study of Black Girls' Vulnerability to Out-of-School Suspensions: The Intersection of Race and Gender." *Children and Youth Services Review* (102): 169–176.

Glaude, Eddie, Jr., interview by Ezra Klein. 2019. "How Whiteness Distorts Our Democracy (and the Ideas That Animate Our Democracy)." *The Ezra Klein Show.* (April 4). Available at https://www.stitcher.com/podcast/vox/the-ezra-klein-show/e/59837986.

Goff, Phillip Atiba, Matthew Christian Jackson, Brooke Allison Lewis Di Leone, Carmen Marie Culotta, and Natalie Ann DiTomasso. 2014. "The Essence of Innocence: Consequences of Dehumanizing Black Children." *Journal of Personality and Social Psychology* 106 (4): 526–545.

Goller-Sojourner, Chad. 2014. "Growing Up 'White,' Transracial Adoptee Learned to Be Black." *Weekend Edition Sunday*. January 26. Available at https://www.npr.org/2014/01/26/266434175/growing-up-white -transracial-adoptee-learned-to-be-black.

Gyekye, Kwame. 1987. *An Essay on African Philosophical Thought: The Akan Conceptual Scheme*. Philadelphia: Temple University Press.

Higginbotham, A. Leon, Jr. 1978. *In the Matter of Color: Race and the American Legal Process: The Colonial Period*. Oxford: Oxford University Press.

Hopkinson, Natalie. 2018. "I Refuse to Give My Black Son 'The Talk.'" *Huffington Post*, September 9. Accessed November 1, 2019. Available at https://www.huffingtonpost.com/entry/opinion-kaepernick-police -brutality-driving-black-men_us_5b9185c2e4b0cf7b003df96f.

Hughes, Langston. 1930. *Not without Laughter*. Alfred A. Knopf.

Institute of Medicine Committee on Understanding and Eliminating Racial and Ethnic Disparities in Health Care. 2013. "Unequal Treatment: Confronting Racial and Ethnic Disparities in Health Care." Edited by Brian D. Smedley, Adrienne Y. Stith, and Alan R. Nelson. Washington, D.C.: National Academies Press.

Karenga, Maulana. 2002. *Introduction to Black Studies*. Los Angeles: University of Sankore Press.

Katznelson, Ira. 2005. *When Affirmative Action Was White: An Untold History of Racial Inequality in Twentieth-Century America*. New York: W. W. Norton.

Kendi, Ibram X. 2016. *Stamped from the Beginning: The Definitive History of Racist Ideas in America*. New York: Nation Books.

———. 2019. *How to Be an Antiracist*. New York: One Book.

Kramer, Rory, and Brianna Remster. 2018. "Stop, Frisk, and Assault? Racial Disparities in Police Use of Force During Investigatory Stops." *Law and Society Review* 52 (4): 960–993.

Levy, Sheri, Steven Stroessner, and Carol Dweck. 1998. "Stereotype Formation and Endorsement: The Role of Implicit Theories." *Journal of Personality and Social Psychology* 74 (6): 1421–1436.

Lopez, German. 2016. "Black Parents Describe 'The Talk' They Give to Their Children about Police." *Vox*. August 8. Accessed June 2019. Available at https://www.vox.com/2016/8/8/12401792/police-black -parents-the-talk.

Marable, Manning. 1997. *Black Liberation in Conservative America*. Boston: South End Press.

McAllister, David. 2009. "Realtors and Racism in Working-Class Philadelphia, 1945–1970." In *African American Urban History Since World War*

II, edited by Kenneth L. Kusmer and Joe W. Trotter, 123–141. Chicago: University of Chicago Press.

Moore, Eddie, Jr., Ali Michael, and Marguerite Penick-Parks. 2018. *The Guide for White Women Who Teach Black Boys*. Edited by Eddie Moore Jr., Ali Michael and Marguerite Penick-Parks. Thousand Oaks: Corwin.

National Center for Education Statistics. n.d. *Fast Facts: Historically Black Colleges and Universities*. U.S. Department of Education and the Institute of Education Sciences. Available at https://nces.ed.gov.

National Women's Law Center. 2017. "Let Her Learn: Stopping School Pushout." *National Clearinghouse on Supporting School Discipline*. Accessed August 28, 2019. Available at https://supportiveschooldiscipline.org/learn/reference-guides/pushout.

Obama, Barack. 2004. *Dreams from My Father: A Story of Race and Inheritance*. New York: Three Rivers Press.

Obama, Michelle. 2018. *Becoming*. New York: Crown Publishing.

Ogletree, Charles, Jr. 2004. *All Deliberate Speed: Reflections on the First Half Century of Brown v. Board of Education*. New York: W. W. Norton.

President's Task Force on 21st Century Policing. 2015. "Final Report of of the President's Task Force on 21st Century Policing." Accessed November 1, 2019. Available at https://cops.usdoj.gov/ric/Publications/cops-p311-pub.pdf.

Simon, Rita J., and Rhonda M. Roorda. 2007. *In Their Parents' Voices: Reflections on Raising Transracial Adoptees*. New York: Columbia University Press.

Smedley, Audrey, and Brian D. Smedley. 2005. "Race as Biology Is Fiction, Racism as a Social Problem Is Real." *American Psychologist* 60 (1): 16–26.

Smith, Susan, Ruth McRoy, Madelyn Freundlich, and Joe Kroll. 2008. *Finding Families for African American Children: The Role of Race and Law in Adoption from Foster Care*. New York: Evan B. Donaldson Adoption Institute.

Spatig-Amerikaner, Ary. 2012. *Unequal Education—Federal Loophole Enables Lower Spending on Students of Color*. Center for American Progress. Accessed November 1, 2019. Available at https://www.americanprogress.org/wp-content/uploads/2012/08/UnequalEduation.pdf.

Spencer, Steven J., Christine Logel, and Paul G. Davies. 2016. "Stereotype Threat." *The Annual Review of Psychology* 67: 415–437.

Stevenson, Bryan. 2015. *Just Mercy: A Story of Justice and Redemption*. New York: Spiegel and Grau.

Sullivan, Shannon. 2014. *Good White People: The Problem with Middle-Class White Anti-Racism*. Albany: SUNY Press.

Tatum, Beverly Daniel. 2017. *Why Are All the Black Kids Sitting Together in the Cafeteria? And Other Conversations about Race.* New York: Basic Books.

Valby, Karen. 2015. "The Realities of Raising a Kid of a Different Race." *Time Magazine*, February 1. Available at https://time.com/the-realities -of-raising-a-kid-of-a-different-race.

Wang, Louise, Corinna Haberland, Cary Thurm, Jay Bhattacharya, and K. T. Park. 2015. "Health Outcomes in US Children with Abdominal Pain at Major Emergency Departments Associated with Race and Socioeconomic Status." *PLoS ONE* 10 (8): 1–17.

Wegmann, Kate M. 2017. "'His Skin Doesn't Match What He Wants to Do': Children's Perceptions of Stereotype Threat." *American Journal of Orthopsychiatry* 87 (6): 615–625.

Wilson, Harry. 2014. "Turning Off the School-to-Prison Pipeline." *Reclaiming Children and Youth* 23, no. 1 (Spring): 49–53.

Index

Dr. Valerie I. Harrison has spent more than thirty years as an attorney, professor, and higher education administrator. She is a graduate of the University of Virginia and Villanova University School of Law and earned her Ph.D. in African American Studies from Temple University. She resides outside of her hometown of Philadelphia, Pennsylvania.

Dr. Kathryn Peach D'Angelo is a lifelong educator with more than twenty-five years of experience as a teacher and administrator. She is a graduate of St. Joseph's University and holds a doctorate in education from Temple University. She resides outside of Philadelphia, Pennsylvania, with her husband, Michael, and their son, Gabriel.

Visit them online at https://dorightbyme.org.